I0476711

0

Internal Medicine

The Guide to Residency

Second edition

Amer Sayed, MD
Augusta University
Internal Medicine Resident

DISCLAIMER

Care has been taken to confirm the accuracy of the information presented in this book by reviewing the literature and books related to the subjects and by including the most common practice information and experience from the authors and editors stand of point . However, the authors, editors, and publisher are NOT responsible for errors or omissions or for any consequences from application of the information in this book and make no warranty, expressed or implied, with respect to the currency, completeness, or accuracy of the contents of the publication. Practitioners are responsible for applying this information into patient's care and the clinical out-come

The authors and editors listed the most common medicine and some of the doses used in practice according to their best knowledge, however, it is highly recommended to recheck the medicine indications and doses from an up-to-date source as they change with time. This is particularly important when the recommended agent is a new or infrequently employed drug. And it is the responsibility of the health care provider to ascertain the FDA status of each drug or device planned for use in clinical practice.

Contact the author by email:
internalmedicinetheguide@gmail.com

Table of Contents

CONTRIBUTORS

All are from Augusta University

Contributing Authors:
All are Augusta University Residents/graduates &
contributed in the following chapters

Eduard Fatakhov, MD
Chapters: 15/19/16/35/2/46/47/51
Haytham Alkhaimy, MD
Chapters: 32/6/3/9/48/7
Scott Graupner, MD
Chapters: 4/1/49/33/8/10
Abhishek Mangaonkar, MD
Chapters: 36/26/27/5/39/25/40
Gita Mehta, MD
Chapters: 34/14/12/37
Sasha Baker, MD
Chapters: 57/30/31

Contributing Editors:
Lee A Merchen, MD, FACP
Program Director, Internal Medicine Residency

James Gossage, MD
Division of Pulmonary/Critical Care
Professor of Medicine

Pascha Schafer, MD
Divison of Cardiology
Associate Program Director

Lu Huber, MD
Division of Nephrology
Assistant Professor

Gyanendra Sharma, MD, FASE, FACC
Division of Cardiology
Professor of Medicine

Thaddeus Carson, MD
Division of Internal Medicine
Assistant Professor

Meshia Wallace, MD
Internal Medicine Resident

Christina DeRemer, Pharm.D., BCPS
Pharmacy Supervisor, Clinical Service (Medicine)

Mike Garcia, PhD
Director of College Composition
Assistant Professor

Medical Students:
Danielle Bayer
Brandon Taylor
Evan Fountain
Amir Makhmalbaf
Zachary Hoffmann
Reshma Reddy
Kunal Patel
Nader Aboujamous

Medical Illustrator
Michael A. Jensen, MS, CMI
Assistant Professor

Special Acknowledgement
Walter J. Moore, MD, MACP, FACR
Division of Rheumatology
Professor of Medicine and Pediatrics

All GRU staff who provided assistance in this project

Preface

This guidebook is written to assist in the transition between medical school and internal medicine residency; it is designed to highlight the most common clinical cases presented and how best to manage them. The topics have been carefully chosen to cover common differential diagnoses to common symptoms. This book will give you a quick summary of what you need clinically to know about them as well as challenges you may encounter in the process. Ideally, this handbook can be read in 1-2 weeks and consulted at any time during residency, but especially during internship.

By reading this guide, written by current internal medicine residents, the reader will benefit from residents' actual experiences, both successes and missteps, which can aid the reader with patient care and case management. The guide includes managing the common clinical problems that patients are admitted for so the intern or the resident will feel confident and display more accuracy in examining the patient, obtaining medical history, writing a thorough and useful history and physical with appropriate work-up.

Unlike the other few available guide or pocket books, this one will NOT address unnecessary and hard-to-remember details you may NOT need in day-to-day practice in order to deliver the most high-yield information in short period of time. Since fourth-year medical students may have only one to two months of internal medicine training, they may become less familiar in managing common diseases after months of training in other specialties (NOT to mention the time traveling during match season and relocation takes). This book will prove to be efficient and effective even during this busy time.

The focus of this guide will be the common explanations for chest pain like acute coronary syndrome, pulmonary embolism; hyper/ hyponatremia, lower/ upper GI bleed, different types of pneumonia, atrial fibrillation, CHF, and so on. The primary resources and references we have used include *Harrison's Principles of Internal Medicine*, the *Washington Manual of Medical Therapeutics*, several published articles on internal medicine, and other resources. This book offers years of experience from residents and attendings, keeping you, a recent medical graduate, in mind. I must reiterate that the input of the attendings who took time to be a part of this project was crucial. This finished guidebook is a culmination of real clinical experience you will encounter presented in an easy-to-reference format written by the fresh perspective and experience of your fellow internal medicine residents.

Amer Sayed, M.D.
Internal Medicine Resident
Augusta University

Foreword

As has been said by many, there is no greater privilege and no more challenging responsibility than to direct the care of those who are ill. More than knowledge, it requires competency, and more than competency it requires virtue, and more than virtue it requires both passion and compassion for another human being in distress. As an internal medicine residency program director for more than 25 years, it has been my joy to observe curious, empathetic, and disciplined students develop into wonderfully compassionate and consummate clinicians. They do this by focusing fully on their patients and their well being as men and women made in the Image of God, rather than data sets. Medicine is much more than making a diagnosis, prescribing a therapy, and offering a prognosis; it is a journey with another soul, sometimes for a shift, a day, a week, or decades.

Dr. Sayed's guidebook offers a convenient roadmap for the beginning of this journey. It is patient, rather than disease centered, and should be used as a starting point for the practice based learning and patient care competencies as well as virtues associated with hospital care and discharge planning. It is compact, convenient, and clear in its approach to the most common symptoms and problems of patients in modern hospitals.

Two things should be recognized by the reader, however: 1) Most hospitalized patients have more than one problem. They have multiple co-morbidities that include multiple diseases, social-economic, and especially psychological and even spiritual complexities that defy simple analysis and interact to thwart simplistic interventions. 2) Situations in which patients find themselves are always dynamic and changing, with a past which may be hidden (especially childhood trauma and abuse), a presence which needs systemic understanding, and a future which depends on timeliness and follow through of plans made.

This reference is a fine start for the genesis of an outstanding clinician. Savvy students will initiate a lifetime habit of frequent and lengthy visits to both the bedside and the enlarging greater body of literature. In each location they will ponder deeply both the causes and the effects of what is happening to their patients. Then, with experience, time, and devotion, they will be able also to taste and give to others the fruits of their practice.

David R. Haburchak, M.D. FACP
Professor of Medicine
Augusta University

Life is short and art long, Opportunity fleeting,
Experience perilous and decision difficult.
                    Hippocrates

Cardiopulmonary

1. Chest pain (CP)

An internist should be able to promptly recognize CP, form a differential diagnosis, & be able to treat accordingly. Remember, the most important part of your assessment is obtaining complete pt hx.

History & physical exam
- <u>O</u>nset
- <u>L</u>ocation
- <u>D</u>uration: just happened few hours ago vs constant for 1 month (later is somewhat reassuring as pt can not have cardiac/ischemic pain for 1 month).
- <u>C</u>haracteristics: Sharp? Achy? Dull? Crushing?
- <u>A</u>ggravating factors that trigger or worsen the CP
- <u>R</u>elieving factors/trial to relieve pain (e.g. whether Tylenol or NTG relieves the pain)
- <u>R</u>adiation: such as to the shoulder, back, jaw, or abdomen.
- <u>T</u>iming of CP: Does the pain wake the pt from sleep? Does the pain occur at rest or when working in the backyard? Similarity to or difference from pain during previous MI (alarming if it is similar to the last MI).
- <u>S</u>everity: (1-10 scale), ever went to zero (w/ like Tylenol or NTG)?

Others: Associated Sx (N/V, diaphoresis, cough, dyspnea, fever, edema, abdominal pain), family hx of cardiac disease or other causes of CP, meds (e.g. ASA, β-blocker, NTG). Also, obtain all cardiac hx such as CHF Sx, chronic angina, smoking, any hx of cardiac intervention or diagnostic tests such as stress testing or cardiac catheterization (including coronary anatomy).

CV	Aortic dissection	Sudden onset of tearing/ripping CP that usually radiates to the back, & may present w/ hemodynamic instability, such as HoTN & tachycardia. Type A affects the ascending aorta (surgical case) while Type B affects the descending aorta (medical case). Control HTN aggressively.
	Acute Coronary Syndrome	Typically ischemic pain is crushing, substernal & left sided CP ("elephant on chest"), which can radiate to the jaw or down the left arm. Associated Sx: diaphoresis, SOB & N/V. If EKG shows ischemic changes or troponin is positive → NSTEMI or STEMI. If EKG shows ischemic changes & troponin is negative → unstable angina (usually >15 minutes). Remember, women & diabetics can present w/ vague non-specific Sx like N/V, so you must be careful in ruling out ACS. If stable angina→ usually lasts 1-5 minutes/ brought on by exertion & or emotion/ relieved by rest or NTG.
	Pericarditis	Friction rub on auscultation, pleuritic CP, EKG shows diffuse ST elevation (down concave) in most of the leads (but ST depression in aVR) & diffuse PR segment depression, pain improves w/ leaning forward (or sometimes just w/ positional changes).
	Arrhythmia	Order an EKG whenever someone presents w/ CP (also consider telemetry).
	Myocarditis	Fever w/ cardiac/CHF Sx. Cardiac arrhythmias is common.

	PE	Acute onset of dyspnea, tachycardia, & tachypnea w/ pleuritic CP (usually w/ pts have risk factors like immobilization).
Pulm	PNA	Pleuritic CP that worsens w/ deep inspiration or cough; can be associated w/ fever, cough, dyspnea, & tachypnea. Dull to percussion & crackles on auscultation.
	PTX	Usually sudden onset of dyspnea/tachypnea, ↓ or absent breath sounds on the affected side.
GI	GERD	Usually postprandial, w/ a burning, gnawing pain, which worsens w/ recumbency. It can mimic cardiac CP (try PPI after ruling out cardiac cause for those w/ cardiac risk factors).
	PUD	Sharp abdominal pain, that radiates from abdomen to chest
	Esoph-ageal spasm	Severe pain w/ eating can be relieved by nitroglycerin. Therefore, it can be difficult to differentiate cardiac origin from esophagus spasm. Tx: CCB
Others	**Costo-chondritis**	Reproducible by palpating the affected area or during chest movement. Pinpoint CP is unlikely to be cardiac.
	Anxiety	Can be similar to cardiac CP in that it can present w/ crushing CP w/ tachycardia, diaphoresis & is brought on by emotional stress.
	HZV (shingles)	Presents w/ a classic rash w/ in a single dermatome. Though during early stages of disease, rash & vesicles may be absent but pt may complain of severe pain in the dermatomal distribution.

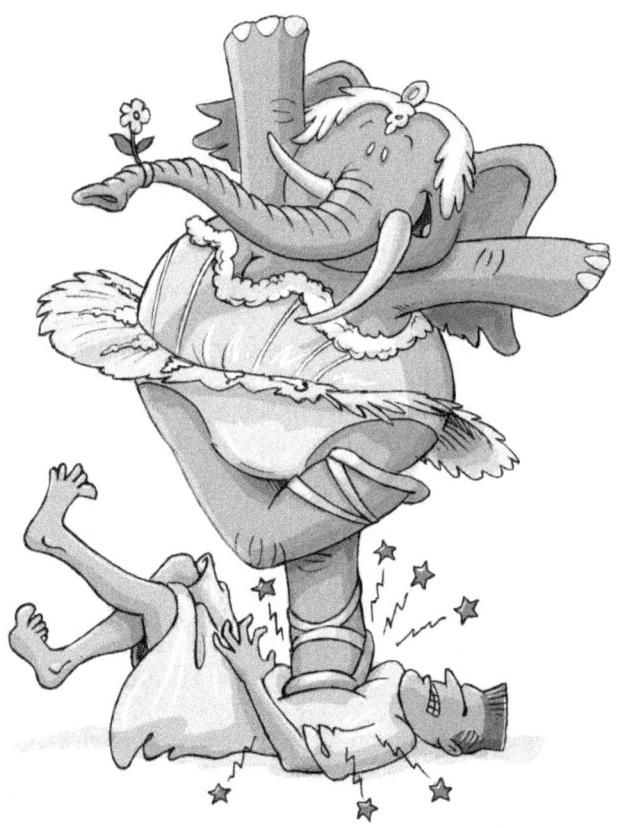

Chest heaviness is typical for acute coronary syndrome.

Management

- Vital signs (ACLS for unstable pt), EKG (compare to prior EKGs if available) & ask above questions (considering the DDx in the above table).
- **If pain appears cardiac in origin,** give ASA 325mg (± Plavix), NTG SL, β-blocker (metoprolol or carvedilol), & Heparin. High dose statins (80mg atorvastatin) are indicated in 24 hours, as well as ACEi like lisinopril in also 24hours as clinical trials

support mortality benefits (NOT in ACS guidelines but recommended).

- Avoid NTG for inferior wall MI because the heart is preload/volume dependent. Also, avoid β blocker if pt is bradycardic (<60). Dual antiplatelet therapy (ASA +Plavix) ↓ mortality especially with loading dose of Plavix (300 0r 600 mg) followed by maintenance dose (75mg).
- Plavix usually delay CABG surgery (or any elective surgery) 5 days due to high bleeding risk until the medicine "wash out" from the body.
- Rule/Out MI or "ROMI" is a common hospital admission for pts w/ CP presented to the emergency department & they did NOT have cardiac enzymes elevation & ischemic EKG changes; regardless of the CP quality (typical or NOT typical for MI). Cardiac enzymes (troponin I) x 3 Q6 hrs is needed for those pts to note the trend (you can also repeat EKGs Q15-30 minutes PRN especially if CP recurs). NSTEMI is diagnosed when troponin is elevated after the chest pain.

> **Attention:** Troponin elevation can happen in some cases, which is NOT related to coronary occlusion like kidney injury (acute or chronic), tachycardia (for any reason like a fib), HTN/HoTN, and infx/sepsis.

- If the troponins continue to show an upward trend, you need to continue trending it until they begin decreasing or at least plateau status.
- Call STEMI code or cardiology "stat" for any chest pain with ST elevation or any other equivalent (poor q wave progression or new LBBB)
- If there are EKG changes, elevated troponin levels, ongoing CP or unstable vitals → call Cardiology. Start the pt on heparin drip w/ a

loading dose protocol, assuming there is no contraindication (weight dose Lovenox is also an alternative to heparin drip, if the kidney function is normal).

Common EKG Changes Seen in STEMI

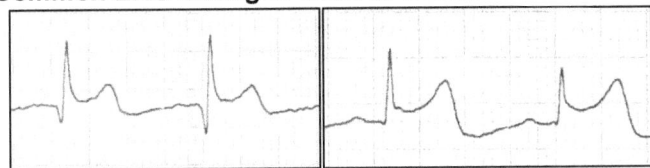

- MONA (morphine, O_2, NTG, ASA) for ACS treatment is outdated & incorrect. O_2 did NOT show benefit unless pt is hypoxic. Morphine may sedate & conceal ongoing ischemia; use morphine w/ caution for chest pain (after NTG sublingual or IV drip for ongoing chest pain). Always use ASA & NTG if NOT contraindicated.
- If pain appears GI in origin, consider PPI or GI cocktail (antacid + Donnatal + lidocaine).
- Always consider the possibility of a PE, pneumothorax, or aortic dissection, as they need very high suspicion.
- If pulm embolism is high on the differential →order EKG (sinus tachycardia), ABG (hypoxia & possible hypocapnia from tachypnea), & chest CTA. Treat w/ heparin drip or lovenox (if NOT contraindicated). If a pulm embolism is somewhat likely, you can obtain a D-dimer assay (low specificity but high sensitivity); discouraged for in pt setting due to low specificity. Consider lower extremity venous US if you suspect DVT & treat w/ heparin/warfarin (or any anticoagx meds) if positive (same Tx as for pulm embolism & hence may NOT need CTA w/o chest pain).
- If PNA is high on the differential, order a CXR, blood/sputum cultures & empiric abx, if appropriate.

- If aortic dissection is high on the differential, obtain a CXR (if hemodynamically stable) to check for mediastinal widening, & consider CTA along w/ vascular surgery consultation as soon as possible.

2. Shortness of breath (SOB)

The subjective sensation of breathlessness commonly referred to as dyspnea.

History
- Is this SOB acute (pulm embolism or PNA), chronic (COPD/CHF), or acute on chronic (COPD/CHF exacerbation)?
- On rest (possible ACS or severe CHF) or exertion (typical for CHF); ask about the baseline SOB, if any, & how worse it is now (how many blocks or feet can they walk?)
- Associated Sx such as cough/sputum (PNA), CP (ACS, PNA), palpitations (a fib or any arrhythmias), fever (PNA), orthopnea/ paroxysmal nocturnal dyspnea PND/ peripheral edema (CHF), legs swelling or weight gain.
- New events or meds near the onset including trauma, IV fluids (pulm edema). Assess adherence to meds.
- Urine output (low in oliguric AKI & severe CHF)

Physical exam
- **Vital signs:** including O_2 sat.
- **Lungs**: respiratory distress, non-labored respirations, accessory muscle use, midline trachea, crackles, wheezes, stridor, egophony, symmetry of breath sounds
- **Cardiac**: JVD (most sensitive/specific sign for CHF), carotids, rate/rhythm, murmurs or rubs, loud P2 (pulm HTN), RV heave (due to RV dilation) & S3.
- **Neuro**: mental status, confused, drowsy (gives an idea of cerebral O_2 delivery)
- **Extremities**: edema, cool vs. warm, capillary refill, & cyanosis (peripheral vs. central)

Work-up

- CXR (check: PNA/COPD)
- EKG (check arrhythmias/sinus tachycardia in pulm embolus/ pulm edema in CHF/ cardiac ischemia)
- ABG (hypoxia in pulm embolus, pulm edema, COPD exacerbation & PNA)
- CBC (Hgb for symptomatic anemia & WBC for PNA)
- BMP (check for AKI)
- BNP (check for CHF exacerbation); >100 is abnormal (>50 for obese pts, unknown why but it is like BNP dissolve in fat).
- Troponin (check for ACS).
- Consider CT angiogram if strong suspicion of pulm embolism (If unable to obtain CT w/ contrast because of kidney injury, obtain a V/Q scan)

Differential diagnosis

- **Pneumonia PNA:** diagnosed clinically. CXR opacities is suggestive (dehydration can delay opacities. If high suspicion, hydrate & repeat CXR), chest CT scan is more sensitive for PNA & can be ordered in complicated picture (very sick pt w/o clear clinical PNA, differentiate between CHF vs PNA vs pulm embolism). Calculate CURB-65 or PNA severity index (estimates mortality, & helps decide where the pt should be treated: in pt, out pt, or ICU).
  CURB-65: all are given 1 point for being present. If pt receives 2 or more points, consider in pt Tx vs out pt; w/ close follow up. If they receive4-5, consider ICU care (online calculator is available & can give estimated mortality rates)
    - Confusion
    - BUN > 19 mg/dL
    - Respiratory Rate > 30
    - BP: Systolic < 90 mmHg or Diastolic < 60 mmHg

- o Age >**65**
- **CHF:** exacerbation (findings: BNP>100/possible pulm edema on x-ray/peripheral edema on exam)
- **MI/ischemia:** dyspnea on rest or exertion can be an angina equivalent (usually SOB is from CHF or lung issues & CP is from ischemia but they overlap).
- **Pulmonary embolism (PE):** common etiology for acute SOB, often difficult to rule in/out by hx/exam. Consider if pt has risk factors; calculate the Wells' Criteria score (online calculator is available). Treat w/ heparin drip/lovenox before waiting for the CTA results (if NOT contraindicated).

> **Attention:** D Dimer testing is discouraged for in pt setting (especially if admitted >2days) due to false positive results.
> In the ED or out pt: Consider D Dimer for low to moderate PE suspicion accordning to Wells's criteria & directly go to CTA for high suspicion (after starting heparin).

- **Pleural effusion:** from CHF vs. Malignancy vs. Infx (x-ray & BNP can be very informative)
- **Volume overload:** from various reasons like CHF or iatrogenic from excessive IV fluid. JVD & LE edema is suggestive & CXR may show pulmonary congestion or frank pulm edema. BNP may be elevated. Stop fluid & diurese (repeat CXR prn to follow resolution).
- **Arrhythmia**: can cause SOB even w/o CHF/ischemia
- **Anemia or anxiety.**
- **Aspiration PNA:** common in pts w/ altered mental status (needs time to show on CXR)
- **Bronchospasm:** can occur in CHF, PNA, & asthma/COPD (trial of jet neb w/ albuterol can help diagnose & treat).

- **Upper airway obstruction:** often acute onset, stridor/focal wheezing (call for ENT evaluation)
- **ARDS:** usually in hospitalized pts & most likely in the ICU (PaO_2 /FiO_2 usually <100)
- **TRALI (Transfusion related acute lung injury):** Usually very rapid onset post-transfusion (usually NOT more than 24 hrs)
- **Pneumothorax:** acute onset, pleuritic CP, consider in intubated pts (especially if peak & plateau pressures are elevated) or post procedures like thoracentesis.
- **Cardiac tamponade:** consider when pt has signs of isolated right heart failure; look for Beck's Triad of Sx ($\downarrow$ BP, distended neck veins, & distant, muffled heart sounds). Check pulsus paradoxus & obtain EKG (should see sinus tachycardia; can see electrical alternans & $\downarrow$ voltage), along w/ the CXR done routinely w/ SOB (if it is large enough you will see a "globular" or enlarged cardiac silhouette on CXR). Have a higher suspicion for this in your dialysis pts, as well as post-cath pts.
- **Others:**
  - **Sepsis**
  - **Metabolic acidosis** (cause tachypnea to blow off CO_2 & compensate)
  - **Massive ascites**
  - **Anaphylaxis** reactions from meds/others (should see signs of edema, urticaria, HoTN); **Tx:** with epinephrine (most important), hydrocortisone, Benadryl, & Famotidine.
  - **Narcotic overdose** can cause respiratory depression, which may NOT manifest as frank SOB feeling due to hypoventilation (give naloxone IV).

Management
1. **Oxygen:** Goal is a PaO_2 > 60 (need ABG), or O_2 sat > 90%. Nasal cannula delivers max FiO_2 ~35-40%, then switch to Venturi mask (delivers up to 50%),

NIPPV (CCU/MICU admission is warranted once pt needed NIPPV; indicate a sick pt needing intensive care). Respiratory Therapist can help w/ nebulizers, suction, masks, ABGs, PO/nasal airways.

2. **Bronchodilator** (Albuterol): Pts w/ wheezing from any etiology can benefit from bronchodilators. All that wheezes is NOT always asthma (e.g. CHF, PNA). Nebulizer: albuterol +/- ipratropium for your COPD & Asthma pts .Use Xopenex for wheezing w/ arterial fibrillation (less β1 agonist effect; less cardiac effect/tachycardia). **In asthma exacerbation:** check peak flows (on PFT) & obtain Gram stain & culture of the sputum.

3. **Lasix**: on pts w/ hx or exam consistent with CHF. Monitor Serum Cr, & be careful w/ CKD pts (they may need higher Lasix doses to diurese). **Diuresis:** double the home dose of Lasix (or any other & give it IV. You can ↑ the dose later if there is still no urine output. Lasix conversion PO→IV is 2: 1 while Bumex (bumetanide) is 1: 1 because it has good bioavailability & GI absorption.

4. **Assess the potential need for intubation** regardless of the SOB etiology (incase of severe hypoxia/ tachycardia). A BiPAP trial may be a helpful method of temporizing while talking to an upper level or waiting for MICU consultation.

- BiPAP is most helpful to correct ventilation deficits (i.e. helps reduce pCO_2), especially in pts w/ CHF or COPD, but can assist any pt to help move air
- BiPAP can be started at 15/5 & can be titrated as needed. Top number refers to IPAP (Inspiratory Positive Airway Pressure) while bottom number refers to EPAP (Expiratory PAP, equivalent to PEEP). You will also need to set the respiratory rate & FiO_2.
- BiPAP is contraindicated in pts who are at risk of aspiration, on tube feeds, have excessive secretions, AMS, or respiratory arrest

(remember the contraindications to BiPAP, as
you will see this quite often during your training).
5. Once you have the pt stabilized & have the results of
your initial studies, you can initiate therapy directed
at the specific etiology of the pt's dyspnea.

3. Congestive heart failure (CHF)

CHF pts usually present w/ SOB, particularly on exertion, mostly from volume overload & ↑ intra-ventricular filling pressures & can present with:

- **SOB or DOE**
- Generalized or lower extremity **edema**/ascites & weight gain,
- **Rales** on lung examination due to pulm congestion/edema,
- **Orthopnea** (ask how many pillows pt uses), & **paroxysmal nocturnal dyspnea** (PND).
- **Jugular venous distention** (JVD)
- **S3 gallop** on heart auscultation,

Two CHF types
1. **Systolic:** which is predicted by reduced EF (normal >55%)
2. **Preserved EF (or diastolic):** when the EF is normal but the pt has Sx of CHF w/ impaired relaxation. TTE is essential for diagnosis.

Etiology
For ↓ EF CHF: etiology is either ischemic (from CAD) or non-ischemic (broad spectrum DDx but most common cause is HTN). Left heart cath (or stress testing in low risk pts) to assess any reversible CAD is usually the first step in evaluating the cause for newly diagnosed heart failure (out pt process usually/cardiology call).

After ruling out obstructing CAD, then non-ischemic causes can be considered like HTN, structural heart problem (valvular disease), diabetes, obesity, toxins like alcohol (mostly large amount around 5-6 beers a day for more than 5 years), arrhythmias (tachycardia induced cardiomyopathy), volume overload from renal failure (insufficient dialysis), anemia, systemic infx, thyroid problems, COPD or pulm embolism (↑ right side afterload), amyloidosis, hemochromatosis, etc.

Preserved EF heart failure
The most common reason is prolonged uncontrolled HTN, & that is why it is sometimes called hypertensive heart disease (LVH on TTE or EKG can give a clue about uncontrolled HTN). Impair relaxation & pseudonormalization (more severe) are echo terms prescribing diastolic failure.

Management
- **CXR:** to check for pulm vascular congestion/edema, effusions, & cardiomegaly (chronic CHF pts may NOT have pulm edema but they still have CHF exacerbation; weight gain & JVD are clues)
- **EKG:** to check for sinus tachycardia, LVH, atrial & ventricular arrhythmia
- **Oximeter +/- ABG:** to check for hypoxia & respiratory alkalosis
- **TTE:** to distinguish systolic from diastolic dysfunction (may NOT need to have new TTE if pt already had one recently & Sx still the same)
- **Labs:** BNP to distinguish from non-cardiac SOB (BNP<100→ low suspicion, BNP>500→↑ suspicion). CMP to check for end organ damage due to hypoperfusion (liver & kidney).

Attention: checking BP is very important at the time of cardiac pulmonary edema presentation, as it will direct the duration/amount of diuresis.

Very high BP w/o peripheral edema may NOT need more than 2-3 liters net negative diuresis (HTN urgency → control BP is the issue) while **normal/low BP** w/ severe peripheral edema (due to maybe diuresis non-adherence) will need much more diuresis (fluid overload is the issue)

Acute treatment

Acute pulm edema is a common manifestation for decompensated CHF (diagnosed clinically w/ rales on auscultation/respiratory distress/desating/CXR later) & is treated by **LMNOP:** Lasix IV, Morphine PRN (w/caution due to sedating effect), Nitrates, O_2, & Position (sitting up on the bed to ↓ preload) along w/ maximizing CHF meds.

> **Attention:** controlling heart rate and BP is essential for pts w/ diastolic dysfunction as well as keeping them Euvolemic w/diuresis.

Chronic treatment of systolic dysfunction (EF <50%) is based on the use of **ACE inhibitors, β blockers, hydralazine w/ isosorbide dinitrate & spironolactone. Diuretics** are also used but have NOT been proven to lower mortality. **Digoxin** is used to ↓ Sx & ↓ frequency of hospitalizations but has NOT been shown to ↓ mortality. **ACE inhibitors** can be used interchangeably w/ **ARBs.** The two common **β blockers** w/ evidence for lowering mortality in CHF are metoprolol & carvedilol (Bisoprolol does but NOT commonly used). ACE inhibitors & β blockers are indicated for CHF pts w/ systolic dysfunction at any stage of disease. **Spironolactone** lowers mortality for more advanced, Symptomatic disease, NYHA III-IV (should be added after maximizing β blocker & ACEi/ARB doses). Eplerenone is also K sparing diuretic, which is specifically good for CHF post MI (↓ mortality). Any pt originally presenting w/ pulm edema should get spironolactone.

Consider **intracardiac defibrillator (ICD)** when EF is <35% (for non-ischemic & <30% for ischemic cardiomyopathy) for more than 3 months on optimal medical Tx to prevent possible serious arrhythmias (mortality benefit due to primary prevention). ICD for primary prevention is usually an out pt process (when life expectancy is >1 year). If EF improved from reperfusion (from stents or CABG) or optimal medical therapy → no need for ICD.

Chronic treatment of diastolic dysfunction (preserved EF) is reliably treated w/ **diuretics.** However, you have to be careful NOT to overuse them. Benefit of β blocker & ACE inhibitors for diastolic dysfunction is NOT clear but they can be used to control BP (on rest & exertion) & heart rate (especially in case of A fib). Digoxin & spironolactone definitely do NOT help diastolic dysfunction (as for now but investigations are ongoing)

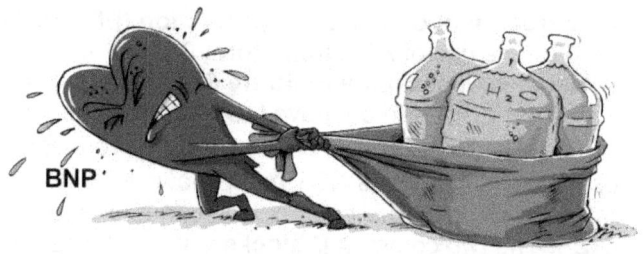

Heart failure (systolic/diastolic) is most often a struggle w/ fluid overload. Assess fluid status & diurese as needed.

Special consideration
- Left & right CHF is another heart failure classification. The left CHF is the common one & it can cause consequently right HF. Right HF can be the primary problem & manifest as LE edema, hepatocongestion, hepatojugular reflex, & ascites. Common etiology is pulm HTN, which can be assessed better by TTE or even right

cardiac cath (to assess pulm artery resistance & effectiveness of Tx w/ med like sildenafil).

- Common **CHF exacerbation triggers** is non-compliance w/: meds (especially diuresis), low Na diet, fluid restriction, adjusting diuretic doses to the daily weight, dialysis (ESRD pts on dialysis). Another triggers: acute illness/infection, ischemia & iatrogenic (meds changes).
- "**Quick assessment" for CHF**: assess volume status, "wet or dry" to direct your diuretics management (like pulm edema, peripheral edema & JVD) & assess perfusion status "cold or warm" to direct your admission to the floor or ICU (extremities temperature, peripheral capillary perfusion). For "cold & dry or cold & wet", admit to the ICU for possible inotropic drip (like milrinone).
- For in pt management of **acute CHF exacerbation**, we generally start diuretic therapy w/ IV furosemide for 24-48h & then switch to PO form (& discharge when pt is Euvolemic). Consider switching to torsemide or bumetanide if the response to furosemide is inadequate. We can also try to use metolazone w/ loop diuretics (usually 30 minutes before the loop diuretics) to treat refractory edema because of the synergistic effect (monitor Mg & K closely). Always have a target for diuresis & urine output to achieve net fluid balance of negative ~1L/day & titrate the diuretic dose up & down accordingly. Consider HD/ultrafiltration to take fluid off for ESRD pts w/ CHF (as most of the time they do NOT make urine).
- Note that in pts w/ chronic kidney disease, ↓ glomerular filtration rate (GFR) is associated w/ ↑ plasma BNP. Also note that obese pts tend to have "pseudo" lower plasma BNP than non-obese pts (BNP dissolve in fat). Do NOT follow up BNP results to direct diuresis (did NOT show

to help). Get BNP just on admission & before discharge (BNP when pt is almost dry/Euvolemic for comparison in the future).

- If a pt presents w/ CHF exacerbation & is already on β blocker, you should ↓ dose by 50% temporarily in the acute phase; & if NOT on β blocker, you do NOT start it until the acute exacerbation resolves.
- Metoprolol succinate & Carvedilol (cheaper) are equal efficacy for LV dysfunction (↓ EF). Sometimes BP is at the low normal (like 100s, systolic) & Pt can NOT tolerate Coreg (due to alpha antagonist effect). In this scenario metoprolol will be a good alternative.
- **All CHF pts need close follow up** by cardiology or PCP W/ in 1 week to evaluate volume status & reconcile meds (as hospitals will NOT be reimbursed for readmission w/in 30 days from discharge). They also need to weigh themselves & call their doctor if there is weight gain more than 2-3lbs in 2days or 5lbs in 1 week (or pt simply can ↑ their diuresis dose as instructed like taking an extra tab) as intervention when these conditions are met has shown improved survival.
- **Pts w/ end-stage refractory CHF** (on optimal meds w/ NYHA class III- IV & >2-3 CHF admissions in 6 months) are candidates for extraordinary forms of therapy (LVAD or heart transplant) or for compassionate end-of-life care due to poor prognosis. High-risk feature for CHF: tachycardia, HoTN, worsening kidney function, ↑ liver enzymes/coagulopathy, ↑ lactic acid & AMS.

- **New York Heart Association NYHA** to assess exercise intolerance to know the severity of the CHF & direct the Tx.

Class 1	No physical limitation from CHF
Class II	Sx w/ ordinary activity (mild)
Class III	Sx w/ less than ordinary (minimal) activity like walking short distance or changing clothes but NOT on rest (moderate)
Class IV	Sx on rest (severe)

CHF Sx: fatigue, palpitation, dyspnea, or anginal pain.
Ordinary activity: is what a healthy person able to do like running, walking, climbing stairs, etc w/o CHF Sx.

4. Coronary Artery Disease (CAD)

The #1 cause of death in the USA & the world.

Cause

Atherosclerotic plaques in coronary arteries w/ some degree of obstruction. Usual intervention is w/ balloon/stents/CABG for lesions or stenosis>70% of the lumen of a large artery (LAD, RCA, diagonal, etc). Coronary ischemia is due to an imbalance between blood supply & O_2 demand, leading to inadequate perfusion.

Risk factors

Elevated LDL, ↓ HDL, smoking, HTN, DM, renal disease (especially Hemodialysis), genetics (family hx, especially 1st degree relative of male <55 or women <65), age (men over 45, women over 55), obesity, & sedentary life style.

Symptoms

Chronic or stable angina usually occurs w/ exercise or emotion (usually lasts <15 minutes & is relieved w/ rest or nitroglycerin). Typical Ischemic CP can be associated w/ SOB (most common), N/V, diaphoresis, & radiation of pain to left arm, neck or scapula. Unstable angina (consider ACS) occurs at rest (& also if the angina is new or ↑ chronic angina frequency/severity→ unstable angina). CAD (especially >60 years old) have no active Sx (which means that the lesions are NOT large enough to cause Sx usually >70% stenosis but they are still at risk of plaque ruptures & STEMI). For full work up of CP please see chapter under CP.

Diagnosis

- **Resting EKG:** look for Q waves (prior MI), any ST segment or T wave abnormalities, R wave progression & new AV blocks (new LBBB is

STEMI equivalent). Normal EKG during the chest pain is maybe reassuring but still does NOT r/o ACS (it is better to have more than one EKG; w/ & w/o CP). Make sure that the EKG changes are new comparing to a previous one as most of EKG ischemic changes can be normal variants if they are existed on previous ones

- **Exercise stress test** (if capable of walking on treadmill for 5-10 minutes): stress EKG or stress TTE. Stress test should NOT be done in the acute setting. Either at the same hospitalization (after r/u MI) or in few days after discharge as an out pt (in case of risk factors & moderate pretest probability for CAD)
- **Pharmacological stress test** for those who can NOT tolerate exercise stress test: IV adenosine, dipyridamole, or dobutamine can be used as cardiac stress inducing agents, which can be combined w/ an EKG, TTE, or Nuclear Perfusion Imaging.
- **Percutaneous Coronary Angiography PCA**: most sensitive test, used in pts being considered for revascularization (Percutaneous Transluminal Coronary Angioplasty (PTCA) or Coronary Artery Bypass Grafting (CABG)

Management
- Please refer to chest pain chapter for the **acute management.** Below is the chronic management, including secondary prevention.
- **Lifestyle modifications:** smoking cessation (can cut risk of CAD in half one year after smoking cessation), weight loss, diet & exercise (reduced intake of saturated fats & cholesterol)
- **Blood pressure control** in pts w/ HTN, goal: <130/90
- **Strict glycemic control** in pts w/ DM, goal A1C <6.5 (unless elderly w/ multiple comorbidities & risk for Hypoglycemia, goal A1C 7-8).

- **Medical therapy:** ASA, β blockers, Ca channels blockers, Statins, as well as Nitrates (either short acting like NTG tab/spray or long acting like Isosorbide mononitrate –Imdur-). In pts w/ recent stent placement, make sure they are taking additional ADP platelet receptor blocker such as Plavix (clopidogrel) or Effient (prasugrel) for at least 6 weeks (preferred up to 6 months-1year) for Bare-Metal Stent BMS & 1 year for Drug-Eluting Stent (DES).
- **Some lesions are NOT amenable to any intervention** (small artery, very distal, too many, etc) & medical therapy is the only option. End stage CAD is a term for CAD pts NOT candidate for intervention & failed medical therapy to control the CP.
- **Ranolazine (Ranexa):** is a "2nd line" anti-anginal meds for chronic angina & ↑ exercise tolerance by unknown mechanism, which is usually used after using the "1st line" anti-anginal meds (like β blockers, Ca channels blockers, & NTG) with persisting angina Sx. Do NOT use in hepatic impairment & adjust dose in renal impairment.
- **Revascularization** in pts w/ significant (>70%) coronary blockages:
  A. PCA: Coronary stents are now almost universally used in PCI procedures, often following balloon angioplasty, which opens the narrowed artery & facilitates stent placement
  B. CABG: for 3 or more vessels blockage (including left main or LAD) or any lesions are NOT amenable to stents. Some CAD lesions are NOT amenable for PCI or CABG (too many stenosis, no good graft target for CABG, small vessel disease, etc)

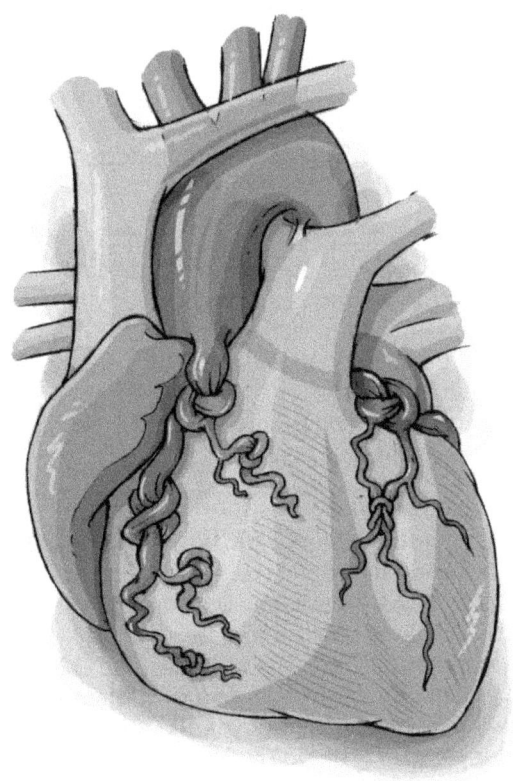

CAD is a common disease. Cardiac disease is the #1 cause of death worldwide.

Special considerations
- **Women & diabetics usually present w/ atypical symptoms** like N/V, abdominal pain, SOB or just generalized fatigue. Do NOT think about ACS only w/ CP.
- **Rule out MI** is a general term for pts who present w/ typical or atypical CP but they have negative troponin x1 & EKG is NOT ischemic. Admission may be warranted for observation to r/o ACS by serial troponin (usually q6hrs) & EKG

(if CP reoccur). Starting heparin drip or weight base dose lovenox is may be indicated for pts w/ high suspicion of ACS (like hx of MIs, typical CP, multiple risk factors, etc). Sometimes pts w/ low suspicion of ACS are admitted for serial troponins & EKG w/o starting heparin (depends on clinical judjement)

> **Attention:** Some pts has significant incompliant history w/ meds or diet or physician visits; placing Drug Eluting Stents DES is may be very dangerous due to the in-stent stenosis & thrombosis risk if they did NOT take palvix (medical management is better than stents; no need for heart cath).

- **Demand ischemia (or type 2 NSTEMI)** manifest by troponin elevation w/o plaque rupture (& intracoronary thrombosis like in ACS which is usually treated by heparin/balloon/stents). ↑ Cardiac O2 demand which results by ischemia occur in: sepsis, any infx, bacteremia, tachycardia for any reason, severe HTN or HoTN, Hypoxia or anemia (& basically anything will cause "cardiac stress"). **No indication (most of the time) for urgent PCA, especially w/ an active infx.** Although demand ischemia is well known but it is somewhat hard to diagnose & based on speculation; some pts will still have heart cath & it will be non-obstructive (usually troponin elevation is NOT very high, <1). **Prognosis:** is still poor w/ any troponin elevation even w/o coronary obstruction/thrombosis (↑ mortality similar to the "real" NSTEMI, type 1).
- **Cocaine:** do NOT start & even stop β blockers in case of cocaine use (contraindicated due to refractory HTN). The use of β blockers may exacerbate the vasospasm induced by cocaine

due to an "unopposed alpha 1 effect" which may cause a significantly elevated systemic blood pressure.

- Around 40% of sudden death from ACS occurred from **plaque rupture** in pts with even 30-50% stenosis "non-obstructive lesions" which do NOT indicate PCI (balloon/stents). Therefore, 90% lesions (which may cause angina symptoms) may NOT cause mortality as the 30% lesions as the later has higher % to rupture due to the high blood flow status, which can cause fibrous cap erosion and, subsequent, rupture. This makes the whole preop evaluation & risk stratification maybe questionable.

- **Anginal equivalent:** acute induction or worsening of diastolic dysfunction by ischemia raises left atrial & pulm venous pressure. This explains why many patients with coronary heart disease have respiratory symptoms with their anginal pain, including wheezing, an inability to take a deep breath, SOB, & even overt pulm edema. These respiratory symptoms can occur in the absence of anginal pain & are often referred to as **"anginal equivalents."**

- **TIMI score:** is a very useful tool to assess the risk for ACS (& ask targeted Qs for complete H & P) & help in the decision of "is the CP ischemic or not?" Including TIMI score in your assessment help to quickly estimate the ACS risk.

Age 65 years old or older	1 point
Aspirin used in the last 7 days	1 point
Angina occurred 2 or more times in the last 24 hours	1 point
ST changes 0. 5mm or more on admit EKG	1 point
Serum Troponin or other biomarker elevated	1 point
Coronary Artery Disease history (w/ at least 50% Coronary Artery stenosis)	1 point
Cardiac Risk Factors w/ at least 3 present (e.g. Hypertension, Hyperlipidemia, premature CAD Family History, Tobacco abuse)	1 point

Total score 0-1: 4.7% risk
Total score 2: 8.3% risk
Total score 3: 13.2% risk
Total score 4: 19.9% risk
Total score 5: 26.2% risk
Total score 6-7: 40.9% risk

5. Cough

One of the most common Sx encountered by a physician both in the in pt & out pt setting.

History
The most important question that helps in differentiating the cause of cough is the duration. Other characteristics such as nature of cough or whether associated w/ expectoration are also helpful (wet cough may indicate either viral or bacterial infx). However, sometimes certain clues such as tickling at the back of the nose (indicative of allergy), coughs associated w/ rhinorrhea (upper airway cough syndrome UACS), or cough following an acute illness & associated w/ characteristic inspiratory 'whoop' (Bordetella pertussis) help in identifying a cause. Post-tussive emesis is characteristic for Bordetella pertussis infx (vomiting after continuous cough).

Types
- **Acute (**<3 weeks in duration): Most often due to upper respiratory tract infx & often viral. However, always think of conditions such as pulm embolism, CHF, acute exacerbation of asthma & PNA, which can occasionally present w/ cough. If acute cough is thought to be due to a URI, double-blinded, placebo controlled study supports the use of 1st generation antihistamine & decongestant therapy. A similar study supports the use of naproxen. In infx such as Bordetella pertussis or Chlamydia, early initiation of abx therapy will reduce Sx & hasten recovery, & hence should be always considered in the differential (Tx: Z pack).
- **Subacute** (3-8 weeks in duration): Should be classified into two groups, (i.e. related to infx or not). Many times, cough lingers on after a URI, suggesting a post-infectious etiology. Bordetella pertussis should always be in the differential, given its resurgence due to waning effect of childhood vaccine (*Note: In the clinic, please make*

sure all adults have received a Tdap vaccine).
Also, hx should focus on possible allergen or
irritant exposure. If subacute cough is NOT
preceded by an infx, it should be treated as
chronic cough.

- **Chronic** (>8 weeks in duration): Often presents a
diagnostic challenge. It is important to realize that
many cases would have more than one cause.
Also, studies have shown lack of sensitivity &
specificity for questions such as characteristic of
cough or the color of the sputum. The aspects of
hx, which are useful, include duration of cough,
whether pt is receiving ACE inhibitor or whether a
pt smokes or not. A CXR is usually needed to
exclude a specific cause such as a lung mass. If
X-ray is normal, the three most common causes
are Upper Airway Cough Syndrome (UACS),
asthma, & GERD. Also, non-asthmatic
eosinophilic bronchitis (NAEB) should be
considered as well. A lot of emphasis is placed on
sequential empiric therapy, starting w/ UACS, then
asthma, followed by therapy for GERD.

Special considerations

- **Upper Airway Cough Syndrome (UACS):** The
most common cause of chronic cough & its
diagnosis is usually established by complete or
partial resolution following a therapeutic trial of 1st
generation antihistamine & decongestant therapy.
If there is a partial response after about 2 weeks of
initiating therapy, other causes should be
considered, such as asthma. A trial of topical
nasal steroid, nasal anticholinergic agent or nasal
antihistamine can be considered. If Sx are still
persistent, sinus imaging (either a plain film or
sinus CT scan) in indicated w/ initiation of abx.
- **Asthma-induced cough:** If suspicion for asthma
is high, methacholine challenge should be
performed. A positive test usually warrants Tx w/
inhaled corticosteroids & β-agonists. Resolution of

cough may take up to 8 weeks. If Sx do NOT improve, a trial of leukotriene inhibitors or PO corticosteroids can be considered.

- **Non-Asthmatic Eosinophilic Bronchitis (NAEB)**: If UACS & asthma are less likely based on work-up & Tx mentioned above; then NAEB should be considered. Diagnosis is usually established by induced sputum to test for ↑ eosinophil count. Therapy is usually inhalational corticosteroids (trial of PO corticosteroids may be required in some pts).
- **GERD-induced cough:** Pts w/ cough >8 weeks, w/ normal CXR, negative smoking hx, no ACE inhibitor use, who failed to respond to trial of antihistamine & decongestant therapy, nasal or inhalational steroids, followed by a trial of PO steroids usually have GERD-induced cough. Guidelines support starting empiric therapy w/ PPI w/ anti-reflux diet & lifestyle modifications. Prokinetic Tx may be added if there is little response to Tx. A 24 hr esophageal pH monitoring is the diagnostic test of choice.
- **Other causes:** If all tests/empiric strategies fail to reveal an etiology (consider holding ACEi as it can induce cough even w/ chronic use), induced sputum for acid fast staining, bronchoscopy for occult endobronchial tuberculosis, HRCT for bronchiectasis or occult interstitial lung disease should be performed. Other uncommon causes include nonacid reflux disease, swallowing disorder, or CHF.

- **Common cough meds**
1. **Tylenol #3:** controlled meds (w/ codeine; suppress cough centrally)
2. **Robitussin (Guaifenesin):** Treats cough that is caused by colds, flu, or other conditions (expectorant that loosens mucus in lungs)
3. **Robitussin DM:** which is Robitussin plus Dextromethorphan (cough suppressant, act centrally in the medulla like codeine). You can include **Phenylephrine** as decongestant (vasoconstrictor) for URI (symptomatic relief)

> **Attention:** Do NOT "pseudo" treat the cough w/o treating the etiology (if possible).

6. Hypertension (HTN)

Primary HTN

Normal blood pressure		**Systolic <120 mmHg & diastolic <80 mmHg**
PreHTN		Systolic 120 to 139 mmHg or diastolic 80 to 89 mmHg
HTN	Stage 1	Systolic 140 to 159 mmHg or diastolic 90 to 99 mmHg.
	Stage 2	Systolic ≥160 or diastolic ≥100 mmHg

Management
Lifestyle modifications & drug therapy. Consider Na restriction, weight loss, dietary modification, exercise, & relaxation techniques. If lifestyle modifications have no effect over 3-6 months→initiate medical therapy (initiate meds if stage 2 directly)

Tx:
Consider comorbidities & drug adverse effects (DAE):
- **Thiazide diuretics** such as HCTZ or chlorthalidone (better than HCTZ) are very common. DAE: hyponatremia, ↑ Ca reabsorption (prevent osteoporosis) & ↑ uric acid reabsorption (worsen gout) in the kidney.
- **Diabetes:** use ACE-I/ARB (like lisinopril/losartan) as it protects the kidney & helps w/ proteinuria. DAE: AKI (in pts w/ CKD), ↑ K, cough, angioedema (tongue/throat/face swelling w/ SOB). Do NOT use if Cr>2. 5-3 or in renal artery stenosis. Monitor BMP (Cr & K) more frequent

when you first start ACEi/ARB (↑ in Cr <30% of baseline is expected due to the mechanism of action & meds should NOT be stopped just because of that). ACEi/ARB are contraindicated in pregnancy (do NOT prescribe if pt is trying to conceive, category D)

- **CAD:** use β blocker (metoprolol either short acting like titrate q12h or succinate q24h, atenolol, Coreg)
- **CHF:** use β blocker, ACE-I or ARB (if ACE-I is NOT tolerated, use ARB)
- **Migraine:** β blocker or CCB (it has prophylactic effects)
- **Hyperthyroidism:** β blocker (Propranolol)
- **Osteoporosis:** thiazide (because it reabsorbsCa) & avoid thiazide in gout (reabsorbs uric acid)
- **Pregnancy:** alpha methyldopa, labetalol, CCB, Clonidine (rebound HTN is common in case of sudden stoppage), thiazide diuretics & hydralazine (used IV for preeclampsia)
- **BPH:** alpha blocker (Prazosin or flomax)

If BP is NOT controlled w/ one drug, add a second drug: β blocker, ACE-I/ARB, CCB, sprinolactone, thiazide
If BP is still NOT controlled w/ the second drug, add a third drug (include diuretics if NOT already) & investigate for secondary HTN causes (preferably after 24 hrs continues BP monitor to confirm elevated BP).

Secondary HTN
Investigate for secondary HTN if you see the following: Young (<30) or old (>60) pt, refractory HTN (failure to control w/ 3 meds including diuretics), Bruit (renal artery stenosis), Episodic HTN (pheochromocytoma), Buffalo hump, truncal obesity, striae (Cushing's), Hypokalemia (Conn's), UE pressure>LE pressure (coarctation of the aorta), & Hirsutism (congenital adrenal hyperplasia)

Special considerations:

- **Start w/ two anti HTN meds** for pts w/ Stage 2 HTN & adjust doses in following visits (usually one med is NOT enough).
- **Check BP multiple times** (do NOT diagnose HTN from single reading), no caffeine, empty bladder, no tobacco or EtOH, relaxed, sitting down & try different devices if error suspected (or manually).
- **Every effort should be done to put pts on β blocker & ACE-I/ARB** due to the great mortality benefits they offer to diabetic & CHF pts. Escalate the doses as tolerated & check the heart rate for the β blocker (do NOT escalate if HR around 60) & the serum Cr for ACE-I.
- **Elderly Pts** especially w/ long-term DM & ESRD (stiff arteries due to calcification) experience hypotensive Sx on normal systolic BP readings like 110s-120s. De-escalate BP meds to achieve "new normal BP" in the range of 140s-150s.
- **HTN Emergency:** BP >210s/120s w/ end organ damage (like AMS, AKI, elevated liver enzymes, pulm edema) needs immediate action w/ IV drip meds like NTG, Na nitroprusside, Labetalol/ Esmolol, Nicardipine & fenoldopam. PO meds can also be used like Hydralazin &/or Clonidine while waiting for the drip.
- **HTN urgency** (same as emergency but no end organ damage) can be managed on the floor w/ PO agents like nitropaste (topical), hydralazine, Clonidine, captopril (short acting NOT lisinopril which is long acting) & labetalol. Do NOT ↓ BP more than 25% in the 1st 6 hrs (could cause cerebral hypoperfusion). Non-compliance w/ HTN meds (especially Clonidine & β blocker) is a common reason for extreme HTN.
- **Elevated BP can be caused by CNS problems** like CVA or elevated intra-cranial pressure (ICP). Do NOT ↓ systolic BP <140s-150s in the 1st 1-2 days

- **Chronic NSAID** use causes/worsens HTN. Switch to Tylenol if possible.

> **Attention**: decongestants OTC that contain ephedrine could cause worsening HTN →HTN urgency/emergency. Always review new meds for worsening HTN.

- **Thiazides** ↑ serum Ca (& uric acid), whereas **furosemide** ↓ Ca.
- **Controlling BP is very essential** for systolic & diastolic CHF Tx (afterload reduction)
- ↓ **PO intake** is a problem for pt w/ HTN as most of the meds are PO & IV HTN meds is NOT recommended in the floor (mostly in the ICU). Clonidine patches are a good option.

7. Arrhythmias

Very common pathology, it can present as a palpitation feeling or it can be a part of pre-syncope work up. It can be a life threatening event (like V tach) or other common arrhythmias (like SVT, paroxysmal a fib, etc).

Work-up
After asking about the nature of the arrhythmia like: real heart racing or just hear is skipping beats like in PACs/PVCs, how long, spontaneous termination?, pre/syncope? (more serious), ever happened before (how often & if is there any triggers, any OSA Sx (snoring?), any CHF Sx (exercise tolerance & orthopnia?), hyper thyroidism Sx?.

Check: EKG, Holter (if arrhythmia comes on daily bases) or event monitor usually for 30 days (if Sx are less frequent) & TTE (structural heart problem? Like valvular problem or cardiomyopathy). If arrhythmia is detected, consider medical therapy (like β blockers) & /or electrophysiology EP evaluation for possible ablation (more successful on normal heart). Usually arrhythmias are better managed by a general cardiologist or electrophysiologist.

> **Attention:** consider either ICD or life vests if it is a serious rhythm (especially if the Sx are syncope, previous cardiac arrest, or family hx of sudden death).

Diagnostic testing
Like other arrhythmias, EKG/telemetry monitoring (for in pt) & holter/event monitor for out pts who are hemodynamically stable if EKG is normal (detect paroxysmal a fib). Tests for newly diagnosed a fib: TTE (assess heart structures), TSH (r/o hyperthyroidism), Electrolytes (especially K & Mg abnormalities), &

Troponin (ischemia evaluation but a fib is unlikely to be the only sign of ischemia in the absence of other Sx).

Common arrhythmias

- **A. Flutter:** It is managed in the same way as A. fib. The only difference is that the rhythm is regular here (saw tooth p waves). High Success ablation rate (>95%). A fib is discussed separately.
- **Supraventricular Tachycardia (SVT):** many different subtypes (Multifocal Atrial Tachycardia MAT, AV Node Re-entry Tachycardia AVNRT, etc), all are originated from the atrium above the AV node (but AVNRT originates in the AV node), so they are narrow QRS tachycardia (unless conduction delay is present). It has a regular rhythm w/ a ventricular rate of 160-180.
  Tx: Best initial management for unstable pts: synchronized cardioversion.
  Best initial management for stable pts: vagal maneuvers (carotid sinus massage or Valsava; contraindicated if carotid bruit/stenosis is present).
  Next: intravenous adenosine (PS: it should be pushed very fast followed by NS flush because it has a very short half-life, seconds)
  Next: IV metoprolol then amiodarone drip. Shock if refractory.
  Best long-term management: radiofrequency cath ablation (as most of the arrhythmias management, very high successful rate).
- **Multifocal Atrial Tachycardia (MAT):** This condition presents like atrial arrhythmia in association w/ COPD/emphysema (hypoxia). EKG will show polymorphic P waves (HR usually 110-130). **MAT manifests** as an irregular chaotic rhythm on EKG. **Treat** underlying disorder & rate control w/ beta or Ca blockers.
- **Sustained Ventricular Tachycardia (VT):** life-threatening rhythm
  Hemodynamically stable: Amiodarone, lidocaine, or procainamide.

Hemodynamically unstable: synchronized cardioversion & the above meds.

Nonsustained VT (NSVT): lasts for few beats, may be caused by electrolytes abnormality, it can be symptomatic (dizziness, SOB, CP, etc) even if it is NOT sustained.

Tx: Consult cardiology, work up for etiology (mainly ischemia), may need EP study (for possible ablation therapy) especially if no obvious etiology, start β blocker (if NOT contraindicated) & place defibrillator pads/life-vest & consider ICD placement (high% of recurrence if no reversible etiology).

8. Atrial Fibrillation (a fib)

A fib is a tachycardia heart arrhythmia that is important to recognize on monitor & EKG & be able to effectively treat & manage. A fib is either new onset or recurrent. Paroxysmal A fib happens sporadically (self-limiting, intermittent) or persistent (>7days). The main three problems are: Loss of atrial contraction→CHF Sx; left atrium stasis→ thromboemboli; tachycardia→tachycardia induced cardiomyopathy (usually in hours-days)

Common Etiologies of A fib

Hyperthyroid, pulm embolism, Cardiac ischemia, CHF, Mitral valve disease, post surgeries (↑ catecholamine status), Anemia, EtOH (holiday heart), HTN, old age & stimulants (caffeine, amphetamine, cocaine). Try to treat the underlying etiology while treating a fib (if possible).

Clinical features
1. Palpitations, dizziness, angina, or syncope.
2. Fatigue & dyspnea on exertion.
3. Irregularly irregular pulse.
4. CVA (from thrombus embolus to brain)

Evaluation
1. Obtain 12 lead EKG & compare to prior EKG if necessary (old or new).
2. Hx of any previous heart arrhythmias (any palpitations, pre/syncope), hx of OSA, recent surgery or trauma (high catecholamine status).
3. Physical exam: cardiac auscultation (irregular irregularity), check peripheral pulses, JVD, presyncope, DOE.
4. TTE (check L atrium enlaregment, valvular disease, or clots?), & thyroid function.

Management
*   **Check vitals (ACLS for unstable pts).** Unstable pts should undergo immediate synchronized

electrical cardioversion (do NOT wait for TTE or anticoagx). Instability is defined as SBP<90, acute Congestive heart failure, pulm edema, confusion, or CP.

- **Stable pts should have their heart rate slowed** if it is >100-110. You can achieve that w/ rate control meds, which are β Blockers PO or IV up to q6h (metoprolol), Ca channel blockers Po or IV (diltiazem), or digoxin (last resort due to toxicity & low efficiency comparing to the other agents). Consider cardioversion w/ either rhythm control medicine (Amiodarone is commonly used to medically convert the rhythm to sinus & also can control the rate) or electrocardioversion (especially if you want to keep the atrial kick in case of CHF, pulm edema, or HoTN); usually it is a cardiology call. All drips are usually used in ICU setting. **Digoxin:** NOT commonly used anymore but can control the rate only at rest (↑ parasympathic activity but NOT effect sympathic pathway).

> **Attention:** No clear survival benefits from rhytm control (sinus) vs rate control. In general: cardioversion is maybe preferred for 1st onset (better <7days, the earlier the better), unstable, active CHF (to keep the "atrial kick").
> **Attention:** Anticoagulate all pts (regardless of CHADS2 core) after cardioversion for 4-12 weeks as the atria is mechanically stunned and also high risk for recurrence in 1st three months.

- **Acute decompenstated CHF & a fib w/ RVR is a hard combination** to treat as AV blocking agents like β blocker & CCB are needed to control the HR but they will worsening the CHF; call cardiology. **Few options to consider:** DC cardioversion, amiodarone IV bolus/drip/PO (control heart rate as well as ability to convert the rhythm to sinus), & digoxin (IV or PO).

- **Consider Transesophageal Echocardiography (TEE)** to r/o left atrium thrombosis if you want to cardiovert a fib if it occurred >48hours (hard to assess if pt is NOT on telemetry monitoring) & pt is stable (cardiovert unstable pts regardless).

> **Attention:** No need for TEE for pts fully anticoagulated (INR 2-3) for >3-4 weeks. If pt had atrium clots→ delay cardioversion until the clots resolve with anticoagx (to prevent CVA).

- **Check & replace Mg & K** trying to keep Mg above 2 & K above 4.
- **Consider PO anticoagx** depending on CHADS2 score to prevent stroke (risk is usually 3-4% per year & depends on CHADS2 score). Make sure that there is no contraindication like active bleeding or previous recent hemorrhagic strokes when you start anticoagx.
- **AV node ablation & pacemaker:** is a last resort for a fib w/ RVR.
- **CHADS2** is a scoring system to indicate the need for anticoagx & can be calculated as CHF 1 pnt, HTN 1 pnt, Age>75 1 pnt, Diabetes 1 pnt, or Stroke/TIA 2 pnts. PO anticoagx are either warfarin or any of the newer agents like Dabigatran (Pradaxa), Apixaban Eliquis) or rivaroxaban (Xarelto) which are expensive (ensurance companies may NOT cover them). **CHADS2:**
Score 0 → ASA (325mg). Check CHA2D2-VASc to make sure that the score is really low.
Score 1→ either just ASA or ASA + PO anticoagx. Also check VASc

Score ≥2 → PO anticoagx (no need for ASA unless indicated for another reason). No need for VASc as anticoagx is obviously indicated.

- **CHA2D2-VASc:** is another scoring system which maybe better for females (**available online**).
- **HAS-BLED:** is another scoring system to calculate major bleeding risk which can also guide the decision of starting anticaogx for a fib pts (**available online**)

9. Asthma & COPD

Common cause of SOB & DOE associated w/ allergy for asthma & smoking for COPD. Usually wheezing is very suggestive of asthma/COPD.

PFTs findings in pt w/ Asthma & COPD:

FEV1 is ↓ ***& FVC is usually normal*** → ↓ *FEV1/FVC ratio (reversible in Asthma after bronchodilator but NOT in COPD).*

↑ ***in residual volume*** *(more in COPD).*

↓ ***in DLCO*** *caused by destruction of lung interstitium, which is mainly in COPD; especially emphysema (can be normal or high in asthma).*

Exam

Chest (wheezing, PNA signs, pulm edema), heart (CHF signs, gallops, murmurs), extremity (cyanosis, edema, warm), & neurological (AMS from hypoxia).

Management

O_2 & ABG, CXR, Albuterol (inhaled/jet neb) +/- ipratropium, bolus of steroids (usually PO prednisone 40-80mg daily). If fever, sputum, & /or new infiltrate are present on CXR, add ceftriaxone & azithromycin for community-acquired PNA.

Chronic management for asthma

- Start w/ short acting bronchodilator **(albuterol) prn** as rescue meds (for mild Asthma; 1st line Tx).
- If NOT controlled, add a chronic controller meds such as an **inhaled steroid (low dose** or you can step up to **moderate dose** for better control). You can start w/ controller +rescue meds prn if asthma is moderate or severe
- If inhaled albuterol prn & inhaled steroids moderate dose did NOT control Sx (pt is still using albuterol often at the day & wake up at night w/ SOB) add **long acting inhaled beta agonist LABA such as salmeterol or formoterol**. Using

long acting beta agonist w/o inhaled steroid in asthma pts ↑ mortality (but NOT for COPD).
- **PO steroids** are a last resort

Steps in chronic management of COPD
1. Tiotropium or ipratropium inhaler w/ or w/o Albuterol inhaler (as monotherapy)
2. Add long acting inhaled beta agonist LABA such as salmeterol or formoterol.
3. Add inhaled steroids.
4. Add PO steroids (also consider cardiopulm rehabilitation).

For last stages, consider surgical options such as LVRS & lung transplantation.

Attention: LABA can be added before inhaled steroids in COPD pts (but NOT in asthma)

Pneumococcal vaccine & annual influenza vaccine, smoking cessation (improves mortality).
Long-term home O_2 if the **PO_2 < 56** or O_2 **sat <88 %** (improves mortality).

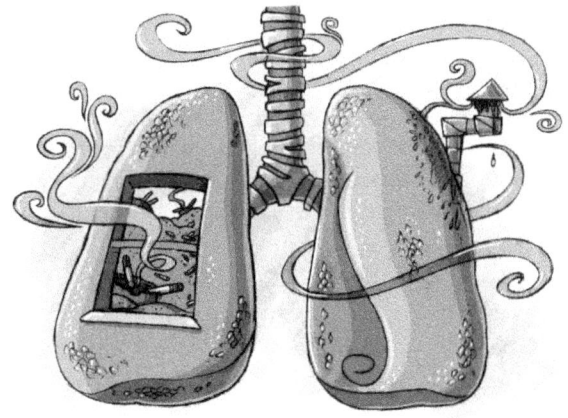

Smoking is #1 preventable cause for COPD.

Special considerations

- Asthma or COPD exacerbation pts who can NOT talk full sentence from their SOB need immediate action by administer O_2 & jet neb (albuterol & ipratropium), IV steroid (methylprednisolone) & possible urgent ICU evaluation (for possible intubation) while awaiting ABG & CXR results. ↑ CO_2 is a sign of imminent respiratory failure from possible respiratory muscle weakness & decompensation.

> **Attention:** β blocker is NOT contraindicated for pts w/ mild to moderate controlled COPD & benefits may out-weigh risks for cardiac indications to use.

- **Consider adjunctive therapy:** like Montelukast or theophylline as indicated
- **Assess severity of the COPD/asthma** w/ FEV1 results: >80% is mild, 80-50% is moderate, 49-30% is severe, <30% is very severe (consider palliative/hospice care evaluation if Symptomatic, on home O_2 & refractory to all meds).
- **Inhaled meds are essential in COPD management;** if a pt is NOT responding to therapy, therapy adherence should be verified & inhaler technique (**available online**) should be assessed before therapy is adjusted (consider spacer to improve inhalation especially for children & dementia pts).

10. Pneumonia (PNA)

PNA is a very common cause for hospital admissions. Knowing how to appropriately recognize & treat PNA is an essential part of internal medicine.

Signs & symptoms
Fever, cough, sputum (yellowish/greenish in bacterial & even viral infx), pleuritic CP, dyspnea, & tachypnea

Work-up
Hx, vitals, physical exam (crackles on auscultation, egophony, tactile fremitus), CXR (infiltration & opacities sometimes are hard to notice & differentiate them from atelectasia), sputum/blood cultures, Strep urine antigen, CBC w/ differential, BMP, & other labs as pertinent (legionella antigen, fungal cultures, respiratory panel, LDH); pleural thoracentesis & bronchoscopy (BAL) if indicated.

Pneumonia Types & Management

- **Community Acquired Pneumonia (CAP):** Pneumonia acquired outside of medical facility that does NOT fit in the definition of HCAP. Standard out pt therapy is monotherapy w/ a fluoroquinolone (Levaquin) or Augmentin + Azithromycin. In hospital setting, start Ceftriaxone/Azithromycin IV.
- **Healthcare Associated Pneumonia (HCAP):** Criteria include hospitalization in acute care hospital for two or more days in last 90 days, residence in nursing home or long-term care facility in last 30 days, receiving out pt IV therapy or home wound care in last 30 days, or attending hospital clinic or dialysis center w/ in 30 days. Also included PNA that begins 48-72 hrs after hospital admission. Standard abx are Vanc & Zosyn IV (covers G+, G-, & anaerobic including MRSA &

Pseudomonas) as initial therapy. Tailor therapy according to C & S.

- **Ventilator Associated Pneumonia (VAP):** PNA occurring after 48 hrs of pt being intubated & placed on mechanical ventilation. Tx is same as for HCAP (must cover Pseudomonas).

Special considerations

- **Community Acquired PNA Risk Stratification:** good standard guide for admission is **CURB-65:** Confusion, Uremia (BUN >20), Respiratory rate >30, Blood pressure <90/60, Age >65. Score of 0-1: out pt. Score of 2: in pt. Score of 3 or greater: assess for ICU.
- **There are many types of PNA**: bacterial, viral (self-limited/supportive management/Tamiflu in 48hrs), fungal (certain places & immunocompromised pts) causes but this is a good guide for initial management.
- **PNA can be hard to diagnose clinically** for some pts especially CHF pts (BNP may help) & more testing is needed (CXR or chest CT scan). Atelectasis on CXR can look similar to infiltration, which is the cornerstone objective sign for PNA diagnosis. Correlate w/ the clinical picture & do NOT feel obligated to a full course of abx if PNA was misdiagnosed.

> **Attention:** Repeat CXR in 12-24hrs (for comparison) as PNA infiltration unlikely to resolve but atelectasis or fluid edema may do (especially if diuresis is given).

11. Medical Intensive Care Unit (MICU)/Hypotension (HoTN)/Cardiac Arrest

Survival of the critically ill pt depends on initiating life-saving measures in a timely fashion. However, recognizing serious illness before the onset of overt instability can be challenging. For example, younger pts w/ sepsis can appear deceptively well but may develop multiorgan failure w/ in hrs. A systematic approach to pt assessment minimizes the likelihood of delayed recognition of critical illness.

The initial evaluation should consist of a brief bedside hx & focused examination to discern whether immediate action is needed to stabilize the pt's airway, breathing, or circulation. Review of vital signs over the preceding hrs often provides valuable information on the pt's overall current stability.

Common early interventions include intravenous fluid boluses for HoTN, O_2 & noninvasive ventilatory support for respiratory distress, & naloxone or dextrose (D50) for encephalopathy due to narcotics & hypoglycemia, respectively. Studies that may be useful for diagnosing the cause & determining severity of illness include ABG; CBG, Hgb, lactic acid levels, EKG, & portable CXR. Limited bedside TTE to assess the hemodynamic status of unstable pts has ↑ in recent years (i.e.: IVC compressibility).

After imminently life-threatening issues are addressed, a **more comprehensive secondary assessment** should be performed w/ an emphasis on identifying less obvious evidence of organ hypoperfusion. This includes AMS (confusion, agitation), ↓ urine output (<0. 5cc/kg/hr), skin changes (pallor, diaphoresis, cyanosis, cool extremities), & ↑ work of breathing.

Common indications for MICU admission
- Close nursing monitoring (example: unstable vitals for any reason like septic shock), service canNOT be delivered in the floor (like intubation & ventilation, arterial line for BP monitoring).
- Status post cardiac arrest & respiratory failure.
- The need for certain IV infusions (like labetalol, diltiazem, amiodarone, lasix, HCO3, etc).
- Sever physiologic changes (very low or high blood PH, severe electrolytes abnormalities like K, Mg, phosphate).
- DKA & HONK management (until the GAP closes & pt tolerate PO intake & get SQ insulin).
- Urgent /emergent procedures like EGD for (GI bleed) or dialysis (for like sever hyperkalemia or pulm edema).
- Delirium Tremens DT (or EtOH withdrawal needing too much Ativan per CIWA protocol; may need intubation & continuous sedation).
- Severe/ongoing GI bleeding w/ Hgb drop for close monitoring, blood transfusion & possible urgent GI scope (upper or lower).

Reconcile home meds
Thiss an important part of the management after MICU admission (or any hospital admission) & doing your 1st assessment/ work up along w/ initial Tx.

As a general role & due to the critical pt illness, constant ability to monitor the pt closely & the possibility of meds interactions; some meds should be held or switched to other forms.

Some examples:
- **Insulin drip** is preferred (stop PO diabetes meds in general in the hospital)
- **BP meds & diuretics** (hold in septic pts & carefully resume as BP tolerates)
- **Narcotics & pain meds** for chief complaint of AMS, HoTN or any complaints could be from the

meds side effects. AMS is one of the signs of organ dysfunction & it will be clouded w/ those meds on addition of possible HoTN & respiratory failure. Restart meds as appropriate when the diagnosis is clearer & pt is responding to Tx.

- **Psychiatric & sleep meds**: antipsychotic meds like Haldol (1st generation/better in cardiac disease), olanzapine/Quetiapine (2nd generation), & benzos (same reason for holding pain meds; resume as needed). Caution w/ benzos withdrawal seizures for chronic users.
- **Some meds w/ common side effects** like diphenhydramine (for itching; anticholinergic property causes AMS & urinary retention), Baclofen (for muscle spasm; causes AMS)
- **Hold meds which does NOT cause immediate benefits** like statins (if MICU admission is NOT from cardiac etiology), allopurinol, vitamins, etc (to ↓ meds interaction & ADR)

Shock

Shock is a state of ↓ tissue perfusion (mostly from HoTN), which can result in inadequate O_2 delivery for cellular needs (tissue ischemia). Tissues ischemia often results in organ dysfunction if severe or prolonged (usually >30 minutes).

Signs for shock: systolic BP <90, MAP<60, signs of end organ damage from hypoperfusion (↓ urine output, AMS, CP, lactic acidosis from the anaerobic metabolism) & lack of BP response after IV fluid challenge (usually after 2-3 Liters boluses).

Three main types of shock:
1. **Cardiogenic** (massive MI or pulm embolism),
2. **Septic** (from severe infx or anaphylaxis)
3. **Hypovolemic** (severe dehydration or bleeding).

Blood Pressure = Cardiac Output (Heart Rate x Stroke Volume) x Resistance

BP is consistent of few parameters including: peripheral resistance (mainly ↓ in septic shock), cardiac output (mainly ↓ in cardiogenic shock like in MI or CHF but also can be ↓ in septic shock du to the negative cardiac effect from the septic toxins) & preload or blood volume (mainly ↓ in bleeding/ dehydration & even in septic shock → hypovolemia occur due to ↑ capillary permeability & 3rd space loss).

In all types of shock, the therapeutic goals are to support tissues & organs that are dysfunctional or at risk of damage due to hypoperfusion & to restore perfusion if possible.

Perfusion can often be improved by administering some combination of intravenous fluids, vasopressors/ inotropic agents such as:

- **Norepinephrine (levophed):** which is strong α1 agonist (stronger than epinephrine) & β1 agonist (same as Epi)/ moderate β2 agonist (weaker than Epi). "Squeeze" good but **proarrhythmic due to β1 effect**.

> **Attention:** β2 agonist causes HoTN (receptors are in vessels) vs β1 agonist ↑ chronotropic and inotropic effect (receptors in the heart) vs α1 agonist in vessels (NOT in the heart) → vasoconstriction.

- **Phenylephrine**: which is strong α1 agonist. "Squeeze" good but do NOT affect the heart.
- **Vasopressin**: which is a V1 receptor agonist in the vascular smooth muscle of the vessels. Also "squeeze" w/o cardiac direct effect).
- **Dopamine & dobutamine:** less common

- **Epinephrine:** (β agonist mainly).

Understanding the cause of shock & reversing the cause of the abnormal physiologic parameter is the key to successful outcomes. Such directed Tx could include lysis of a massive pulm embolism causing cardiogenic shock or Tx of an infx causing septic shock. If ↑ fluid volume is likely to improve perfusion, intravenous fluids should be given liberally as boluses w/ immediate clinical reassessment (septic pts may need up to 6 liters in the 1st 6 hrs). The adoption of guidelines using physiologic parameters, such as central venous pressure, as targets for resuscitation has improved outcomes by encouraging more timely administration of needed fluids (mostly used is normal saline).

> **Attention**: the adaption of guidelines using physiologic parameters, such as central venous pressure CVP, as targets for resuscitation has improved outcomes by encouraging more timely administration of needed fluids (mostly used is Normal Saline).

Aggressive volume expansion is most important in pts w/ hypovolemic shock & has also been associated w/ improved outcomes in pts w/ septic shock. Concern about precipitating heart failure & pulm edema should NOT modify the need for large bolus volume administration (intubate if needed).

Sepsis

Sepsis is an exaggerated inflammatory response to an infectious stimulus & is characterized by a severe catabolic reaction, widespread endothelial dysfunction, & release of inflammatory agents. The mortality rate of pts w/ sepsis complicated by multiorgan failure may be greater than 70% to 90%; mortality rate can be estimated by adding 15% to 20% predicted mortality for each sepsis-induced organ dysfunction. The term/s:

- **Systemic inflammatory response syndrome (SIRS)** was introduced to describe findings of:
  1. Altered temperature (<36 or >38)
  2. Tachycardia (>100)
  3. Hyperventilation (>20)
  4. Abnormal WBC (<4, 000 or >12, 000) regardless of the cause (inflammatory or infectious).
- **Sepsis** is defined as SIRS plus suspected (or proven) infx (UTI, PNA, cellulitis etc).
- **Severe sepsis** is associated w/ systemic effects including: HoTN, ↓ urine output, or metabolic acidosis.
- **Septic shock** is sepsis w/ persistent organ hypoperfusion despite adequate initial fluid resuscitation, which is usually 30cc/kg (like 3 liters for 100kg pt. That requires vasopressor agents to maintain blood pressure).

> **Attention**: No septic shock w/o persistant HoTN (NOT responding to IV fluid) but sepsis can happen even w/o HoTN.

Management

Treat infx (empiric abx like vanc/zosyn w/ in 30 minutes of recognizing sepsis, if possible) & optimize tissue perfusion (by aggressive fluid resuscitation & vasopressors). Repetitive fluid challenges are performed by giving a 500 to 1000 mL bolus of crystalloid over short intervals while assessing response to target central venous pressure (normal is 8-10, higher number is may be better in case of septic shock).

Most pts need 4 to 6 L of fluid in the first 6 hrs, & a frequent error is underestimating the intravascular volume deficit & the amount of fluid required. Use of crystalloid or colloid is likely equivalent. Vasopressor therapy should be started immediately if the initial fluid challenge fails to restore adequate blood pressure & organ perfusion.

Prolonged hypoperfusion results in worsening ischemia & organ failure. Vasopressor therapy w/ norepinephrine, vasopressin, or phenylephrine is frequently needed to restore perfusion during life-threatening HoTN.

No trials have established a single superior vasopressor agent. Norepinephrine, vasopressor, phenylephrine are 1st-line agents for correcting HoTN in septic shock. Vasopressor agents can be used concurrently w/ fluid resuscitation in life-threatening HoTN.

Being at the upper side of fluid resuscitation is better than under resuscitation & intubate prn if pulm edema & CHF is a concern. Get lactic acid q4-6hrs & monitor the trend; down trending is reassuring & up trending may indicate plan/intervention changing.

Pain, delirium, & sedation in the ICU

- **For pain:** pts in the ICU may NOT be sufficiently interactive to give valid responses. Physiological indicators such as hypertension & tachycardia correlate poorly w/ more intuitively valid measures of pain, but pain scales such as **Critical Care Pain Observation Tool (available online)** which consider facial expression, body movement, vent compliance (for intubated pts) & muscle tension to provide structured & repeatable assessments & it is currently the best available methods for assessing pain. **Tx:** fentanyl IV drip, patches or boluses/morphine IV.
- **For sedation:** it is widely used in the ICU & mostly for intubation. In general, no sedative drug is clearly superior to all others. Sedatives that are commonly used in the ICU: benzodiazepines (GABA agonist) likeVerced (midazolam) & ativan

(lorazepam) vs short-acting intravenous (short-acting & titratable drugs) anesthetic agent propofol, & Precedex (dexmedetomidine; α2-adrenoceptor agonist). Each one has certain benefit & quality. **Precedex have advantages over benzodiazepines**, since it produces analgesia, causes less respiratory depression, & seemingly provides a qualitatively different type of sedation in which patients are more interactive & so potentially better able to communicate their needs (& the best to extubate on if sedation is needed).

- **For delirium:** Delirium is a nonspecific but generally reversible manifestation of acute illness that appears to have many causes, including recovery from a sedated or oversedated state. The pathophysiology of delirium that is associated w/ critical illness remains largely uncharacterized & may vary depending on the cause. Duration of delirium was significantly ↓ w/ early mobilization & interruptions in sedation. **Prevent** w/ Olanzapine (2nd G antipsychotics) & **treat** w/ haldol PO/IV or quetiapine PO (even Precedex drip can be used in hyperactive delirium & showed superiority in some studies over benzos & haldol). Diagnosis of delirium is associated w/ ↑ mortality (estimated as a 10% ↑ in the relative risk of death for each day of delirium). Sedation w/ Precedex rather than benzos appears to reduce the incidence of delirium in the ICU.

Special considerations
- **Assess the need for lines** such as arterial line, central line, hemodialysis line, foley cath.

> **Attention**: short line (like peripheral large lines) are better for resuscitation than long/ narrow lines (like PICC/ central lines) due to ↑ fluid flow resistance with ↑ line length and ↓ line radius.

- **Consider prophylactic meds** like GI ulcers w/ PPI & DVT w/ heparin SQ & check for decubitus ulcers in all ICU pts.
- **Low-dose corticosteroids** as indicated in septic shock refractory to fluids & vasopressor therapy
- **Critically ill pts w/ anemia** who are NOT bleeding & who do NOT have acute coronary syndrome appear to do better w/ more conservative threshold for blood transfusion (Hgb level ≤7 g/dL [70 g/L]) for blood transfusion).
- **Bicarbonate should NOT be used** for the purpose of improving hemodynamics or reducing vasopressor requirement when treating lactic acidosis w/ a pH higher than 7.15.
- **Always consider:** avoiding malnutrition, employing therapist-driven weaning protocols, using sedation protocols w/ a daily interruption in ventilated pts, using intermittent or bolus sedation rather than continuous infusions, & avoiding neuromuscular blockade as possible.
- **Unconscious adult pts w/ spontaneous circulation after out-of-hospital cardiac arrest should be cooled** to 32°C to 34°C for 12 to 24 hrs when the initial rhythm was VF. Such cooling may also be beneficial for other rhythms or in-hospital cardiac arrest. Usually prognosis is poor for pts whom did NOT gain meaningful communication in the next 48-72 hrs (it is better to wait to tell the prognosis to the family until that time pass)
- **Glasgow Coma Scale (GCS)** is a neurological scale that aims to give a reliable, objective way of recording the conscious state of a person for initial

as well as subsequent assessment (**available online**).

> **Attention:** assessing mental status (like s/p code or coma from trauma) should be done "off sedation" which could be needed for intubation or seizure control. No meaningful communication after 3days from the coma (off sedation) has poor prognosis.

- **Sedation holiday** involves stopping the sedative infusions & allowing the patient to be awake. The infusion should only be restarted once the patient is fully awake & obeying commands or until they became uncomfortable or agitated & deemed to require the resumption of sedation. Ideally, this should be performed on a daily basis. This strategy has been shown to ↓ the duration of mechanical ventilation, length of stay in ICU, & ICU delirium w/o increasing adverse events such as self-extubation.
- **Code blue:** ACLS algorithm (**available online**). **As a quick review:**
  1. Unresponsive?
  2. Pulseless?
  3. Start chest compression
  4. IV access/heart rhythm? (place monitor pads) /intubation?
  5. Conisder Elictrical cardioversion (V fib/tach/SVT?), IV meds (epi/HCO3/Mag/IV fluid/amio) prn
  6. Send for basic blood work (CBG, CBC, CMP, lactate, troponin, D Dimer, ABG, etc)
  7. Check the chart, nurse, or primary team for any possible etiology, recent meds or intervention could be related to the code (like high insulin dose or new meds).
  Assess pulse & heart rhythm q2min → check BP if you had **Return Of Spontaneous**

Circulation (**ROSC**) & transfer to ICU. Attempt to call family to update them. **Do not do chest compression on an "awake person".**

12. Acute respiratory failure & basics for oxygen therapy

Respiratory failure results from either hypoxia (low O_2) or hypercapnia (elevated CO_2), or both.

Hypoxemic respiratory failure etiology:

- **Diffusion defect:** ↓ diffusion capacity for any reason like pulm edema & ARDS, **measured by:**
  1. PaO_2 (artrial)/FiO_2 (alveolar) ratio: normal ratio is >500 which is the result of 100 mm Hg dissolved O2 / 21% air O2. The lower the ratio →the worse the defect (the shunt). In severe ARDS the ratio is <100.
  2. A-a gradiet: normal is 4-10 (depends on age too). The higher the gradient → the worse the defect (calculator is **available online** for the two previous ratio & gradient).
- **Hypoventilation:** ↓ minute ventilation leads to ↑ $PaCO_2$ & ↓ PaO_2. **Etiology**: CNS depression, Obesity Hypoventilation syndrome OHS (Pickwickian syndrome), Obstructive Sleep Apenia OSA or Narcotics overdose.
- **Hypovolemia, poor cardiac output, MI**
- **V/Q mismatch:** pulm embolism, Pulm HTN, COPD, Asthma, ILD. Corrects w/ supplemental O_2
- **Shunt:** perfusion to non-ventilated alveoli (collapsed or flooded with fluid, pus or blood) or communication w/ arterial/venous system. From ARDS, PNA, AVM, congenital heart disease, PFO w/ right to left flow. **This does NOT correct w/ supplemental O_2**. Rather, hypoxia is reversed w/ Positive End Expiratory Pressure PEEP support to "recruits" & "open" affected alveoli.
- ↓ **FiO_2 or** ↓ **total O_2** →O_2 replaced by other gases or ↓ O_2 from high altitude

Hypercapnic respiratory failure etiology:

- **CNS disorders/** $\downarrow$ **ventilator drive/drug overdose, OSA**
- **Peripheral nerve disorders:** Guillan Barre Syndrome, ALS, West Nile Virus, ICU acquired myopathy/paresis
- **NMJ disorders:** Myasthenia Gravis, Botulism
- **Muscle disorders:** Muscular Dystrophy
- **Lung:** obstructive lung disease (COPD, Asthma, & CF)
- **Chest wall disorders:** obesity, chest trauma

O_2 facts

- Room Air RA has 21% O_2 (FiO_2 is 21%)
- Supplemental O_2 can $\uparrow$ FiO_2 to 100% (depends on the delivery method)
- 97% O_2 transported to tissues bound to Hgb, 3% dissolved in plasma
- ABG measures PaO_2: pressure of O_2 dissolved in plasma (80-100mmHg is normal)
- O_2 saturation can be measured via pulse ox; normal value >94% (NOT very accurate as it is affected by peripheral perfusion & does NOT tell the CO_2 status, get ABG for better assessment)
- 1L of supplemental O_2 will $\uparrow$ FiO_2 ~3% (like 3L O_2 in facemask will $\uparrow$ FiO_2 to 30%, 21% room air+9%=30%)

Methods of oxygen delivery

- **Nasal Cannula:** can deliver1-6 L/min; FiO_2 24-40%
- **Simple Face Mask:** can deliver5-10 L/min; FiO_2 30-60%. Indicated if pt requires higher O_2 concentration; flow rate can be adjusted as well to prevent re-breathing of exhaled CO_2

- **Non-rebreather mask:** can deliver10-15L/min; FiO_2 60-80%. It has a one way valve which allows exhaled CO_2 to leave mask; ↓ CO_2
- ↑ **flow device:** Delivers O_2 at rates above normal inspiratory flow rate, maintains fixed FiO_2
- **Venturi mask:** can deliver4-12 L/min; FiO_2 24-50%. Uses a nozzle to ↑ O_2 flow & mix w/ air
- **Aerosol devices:** Produce fine mist that can be delivered w/ face mask, tracheostomy (trach) collar or T piece (commonly used before considering extubation to assess spontaneous breathing as it is NOT connected on the ventilator)

Ventilator basics

Non-invasive positive pressure ventilation (NIPPV) , sometimes called "NIV", consists of delivery of positive airway pressure breaths w/o the use of an endotracheal tube or tracheostomy. In general, the interface between the critically ill pt & NPPV device is a tight-fitting mask. It ↓ the work of breathing & results in less energy expenditure to support a pt's required minute ventilation. It is the standard of care for managing moderate to severe COPD exacerbations (to prevent intubation).

Other indications: Cardiogenic pulm edema (treat the edema mechanically until the diuresis work), post-extubation, immune compromised pts (due to ↑ risk for nosocomial infx like intubation associated PNA) & other pts w/ hypoxemic respiratory failure.

> **Attention:** NIV, Non-rebreather & intubation (w/ ↑ RR) are maybe the best interventions to ↓ CO_2.

Contraindications: Severe acidemia, inability to protect airway (in case of vomiting), AMS, aspiration risk, upper GI bleed, impending cardiac/respiratory arrest & Uncooperative pt requiring sedation.

> **Attention**: Non-invasive positive pressure ventilation has the potential to worsen outcomes by excessively delaying, rather than preventing, intubation in high-risk populations. Elective intubation is appropriate for pts w/ acute respiratory failure who do NOT respond to a 1- to 2-hr trial of non-invasive support.

Invasive Mechanical Ventilation: indicated for airway protection & acute respiratory failure, inability to tolerate NIV for above listed contraindications. Modes:

1. **Assist control:** preset tidal volume or pressure. 1st choice in most clinical situations, used commonly for ARDS.
2. **Synchronized Intermittent Mandatory Ventilation SIMV:** delivers preset TV, minimum RR. Spontaneous breathes above minimum mandatory RR triggers variable tidal volume. Spontaneous breaths & mandatory breaths are synchronized to reduce breath stacking/air trapping.
3. **Pressure Support:** Inspiratory pressure support to ↓ work of breathing. Close monitoring required; dependent on pt's lung mechanics.

Weaning

Is the process by which a pt is liberated from mechanical ventilation. Pts are candidates for weaning when they are hemodynamically stable & have recovered from respiratory failure. They should have a cough that is strong enough to clear secretions, a ↓ secretion burden, & a patent upper airway. The rapid shallow breathing index (RSBI) is a method to test the readiness of a pt for weaning & should be measured daily. It is defined as the ratio of the respiratory rate to tidal volume (f/VT). If the f/VT is greater than 105, there is a 95% chance that a spontaneous breathing trial will be unsuccessful; if it is less than 105, there is an 80% chance of success.

Spontaneous breathing trials are usually done by placing the pt on a T-piece where no positive pressure is delivered (only supplemental O_2) or by adjusting the ventilator so that it applies only enough pressure to overcome the resistance of the endotracheal tube. Weaning parameters can be done by Respiratory Therapist (RT) when pt on T-piece →suggest extubation if parameters are good (numbers are **available online**). **Clinically:** if pt is tolerating T-piece for >1 hour once or twice w/o distress like tachycardia & tachypnea (& the original etiology is improving like pulmonary edema or PNA) ± ABG is good →extubate

Daily interruption of sedation (sedation holidays) & spontaneous breathing trials should be used as a standard of care for appropriate pts in critical care units. Their use will shorten the need for mechanical ventilation by an average of 1.5 days, dramatically ↓ the number of pts who require mechanical ventilation for more than 3 weeks, ↓ ICU length of stay, & lower 1-year mortality. Direct extubation to NPPV is effective at weaning pts w/ obstructive lung disease from mechanical ventilation.

Special considerations
- **Positive end-expiratory pressure** is the 1st-line approach to correcting shunt-associated hypoxemia in pts w/ acute respiratory distress syndrome, but it is less applicable in the setting of focal disease.
- **In the intensive care unit:** daily interruption of sedation & spontaneous breathing trials lead to more rapid extubation & lower rate of mechanical ventilation
- **Ventilator-associated PNA** can be prevented by the routine use of protocols that require elevating the head of the bed by 30 degrees & hastening time to extubation.
- **Lung Volumes:** RV: residual volume in lungs at maximal expiration. ERV: air exhaled after normal expiration. TV: air that enters/exits lungs during

normal respiration ~500cc. FRC: functional reserve: RV+ERV. Total Lung Capacity TLC: RV+ERV+TV+ IRV

- **Vent Settings:**
Minute ventilation MV = respiratory rate RR x Tidal volume TV. **RR** usually 12
FiO_2: start w/ 100% FiO_2, then titrate down to goal $PaO_2 \geq 60mmHg$ (or O_2 sat >92%).
PEEP: 5 cm H20 is commonly used; high levels used in ARDS & cardiogenic pulm edema to improve oxygenation. ↓ **TV** (6mL/kg) → ↓ mortality in ARDS.
- **Atelectasis** is an important cause of hypoxemia in surgical (preventable by early use of incentive spirometry before & after surgery) & mechanically ventilated pts.
- The need for large amounts of supplemental O_2 in pts w/ exacerbations of COPD or asthma should prompt consideration of **alternative diagnoses** (as those diagnosis, usually, easily corrected w/ increasing FiO_2)
- **A slightly elevated, or even normal, arterial PCO_2** in a pt w/ an asthma exacerbation may indicate impending respiratory arrest (consider intubation). Pts w/ a severe asthma exacerbation that does NOT respond to 1 hr of aggressive bronchodilator therapy are candidates for admission to the intensive care unit.
- **Pts w/ acute upper airway obstruction (like in angioedema) should be closely monitored** & low threshold for intubation should be considered given the difficulty of endotracheal tube placement in this population. Consider ENT consult for laryngeal scope & MICU evaluation for Angioedema pts (pt on lisinopril w/ lips/tongue sudden swelling/hoarseness) even if they do NOT look in respiratory distress at the time of presentation due to the high risk of sudden deterioration.

- **The physiologic hallmark of ARDS is acute (<1week) hypoxemia:** (w/ bilateral infiltration w/o other lung pathology like nodules/pleural effusion or cardiac pulm edema), which is typically corrected w/ mechanical ventilation combined w/ supplemental O_2 & positive end-expiratory pressure. In pts w/ ARDS, limiting tidal volumes, minimizing plateau pressure, optimizing positive end-expiratory pressure, & reducing FIO_2 to less than 0.6 may help prevent ventilator-associated lung injury. Usually ARDS recovery/Tx is long (if pt recovers in 2-3 days →not ARDS)
- **Hypercapnic:** is tolerated much better than hypoxia
- **"Trach collar"** is a term to describe pts who had tracheostomy & on ventilator (for maybe pressure support)
- **"Weaning on sedation":** is maybe useful for anxious pts, especially if the parameters & ABG is good on T-piece trials (anxiety from feeling thy can NOT breathe independently from maybe long mechanical ventilation).

13. Cardiology diagnostics & interventions

EKG:

Is better to be reviewed in a systemic way:

- **P wave in lead II:** upright; means sinus mechanism (tell you that the signal is generating from the sinus node going toward AV node along with lead II axis, it can still be abnormal)

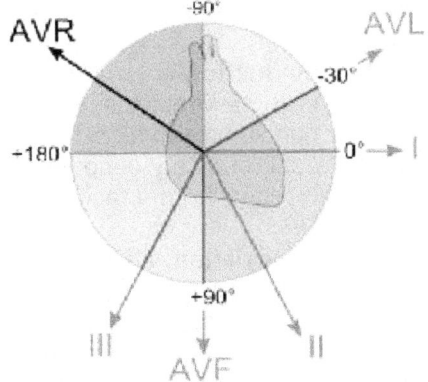

- **PR interval:** normal from 0. 12 - 0. 2 sec (one square is 0. 04 sec). **PR>0. 2 sec→** block → **1ˢᵗ degree block**: PR interval is the same throughout
  2ⁿᵈ degree block, mobitz one,: increasing in PR interval w/ a drop in QRS (small PR then longer & longer until one P wave does NOT conduct through AV node & no QRS following)
  2ⁿᵈ degree block, mobitz two,: fixed prolonged PR w/ dropped QRS (the same prolonged PR throughout for few beats until one P w/o QRS).
  3ʳᵈ degree heart block: P waves are dissociated from QRS. P is NOT conducting through AV node → Escape rhythm →narrow QRS (AV junction) or

wide QRS (below AV junction→ ventricular rhythm which is usually slower than junctional)
The last 2 blocks are advanced blockages & may NOT be reversible (need PPM). Short PR interval (<0.04 sec) could indicate an accessory pathway (look for delta wave –wolf parkinsons white-).

- **P wave morphology** (should be the same if originating from the same focus & different if from several sites). PP interval should be the same if originating from the same focus.
- **QRS:** narrow (depolarization starts from atrium or close to AV node/junctional) or wide >0. 12 sec (when depolarization from ventricle or RBBB/LBBB).
  Aberrant conduction is usually an intermittent wide QRS in supra-ventricular tachycardias due to temporary bundle branch blocks (usually RBBB due to different refractory periods). Sometime it is hard to recognize it from V tach (wide QRS tachycardia).
- **ST segment deviation:** elevated w/ upward concavity (in STEMI, pericarditis, CNS etiology, normal variant) or depressed (NSTEMI, demand ischemia, LVH, digoxin, normal). Recognizing early depolarization as a normal variant is essential (up-sloping STE may be a normal variant, horizontal or down sloping is always concerning).
- **T wave abnormalities:** inversion (from ischemia, hypokalemia, or normal variant), peaking (hyperkalemia), flattening/biphasic (ischemia or non-specific).
- **R wave progression:** normally, R wave progress in V leads from 1 to 6. Failure to progress may be a sign of ischemia/STEMI (or old MI, LBBB).
- **Pathologic Q wave:** >30 msec or >25% height of the R wave in that complex. Normal if smaller (septal depolarization).
- **QT prolongation** (>440msec): calculate QTc (**available online**), depends on heart rate & sex.

- **Rate:** 300/large square# between RR (tachycardia>100 & bradycardia <60).
- **Axis:** normal (QRS is positive in leads I & II), right (QRS is negative in lead I), or left (QRS is negative in leads II & III).
- **LVH:** either R >11 small squares in lead AVL or R in V5 or V6 pulse S in V1 is more than 35mm
- **RVH:** R>S in V1 or R >7 mm in V1, S in V5 or V6 >7 mm.

Attention: Wide complex QRS does NOT automatically means → ventricular rhythm. That is especially important when you have SVT tachycardia w/ abberant conduction
(NOT V Tach).

Special considerations
- **Always compare the EKG** to a previous one (if available) to check for changes & to make sure any abnormality was NOT already present before.
- **Wide QRS** can be from ventricular rhythm (ventricular tachycardia/fibrillation or ventricular escape rhythm if SN is dysfunctional → no P or AV node is NOT conducting → P is present but NOT conducting), RBBB (RQRȯin V1), or LBBB (wide Q wave in V1/poor R wave progression).
- **Ischemic ST elevation is convex** (NOT upwards).
- **Ischemic ST depression is horizontal or down-slopping.**
- **In old infarction, Q wave is wide & deep** (NOT small as in septal depolarization normal Q wave) & T wave can be upright or inverted on the same lead.
- **QRS is a mirror image** in V6 & lead I in LBBB.
- **Ventricular tachycardia & fibrillation are shockable** rhythms, especially if hemodynamically unstable.

- **Caliber is very essential** in reading an ECG to measure the PP interval & QQ interval.
- **Ectopic beats:** random scattered QRS, which could be from atrium (narrow) or ventricle (wide).

Trans-Thoracic Echocardiogram (TTE)
Noninvasive, easy, & very informative procedure to assess the heart structure including:
- **Valvular abnormality**: stenosis & regurgitation (heart "tolerate" regurgitation more than stenosis),
- **LVH**: sign of long-term uncontrolled HTN.
- **RVH:** sign of long-term elevated pulm HTN for any reason.
- **Chamber enlargements:** like atriums enlargement from valvular disease. This enlargement can cause **a fib** from pulmonary veins stretching in left atrium → surgery is a last resort (MAZE procedure or Pulmonary Vein Isolation PVI)
- **Wall-motion abnormalities (WMA):** hypokinesia or akinesia, may be a sign of new ischemia if new & localized to one region such as inferior or anterior wall. It can be reversible in stress echo test which may indicate ischemia (irriveresible in old infarction)
- **Ejection fraction**: very accurate non-invasive test for EF. Left heart cath is invasive but more accurate in EF estimation & usually is 5-8% higher than the other tests like TTE, nuclear or MRI).
- **Diastolic function**: impaired relaxation (milder) & pseudo-normalization (worse)→ CHF w/ preserved EF.
- **Pulm pressure**: elevated in lung pathology like COPD, OSA, or from left pathology such as LV dysfunction or MR/MS or even idiopathic/ right heart cath is more accurate & needed in case of pre-liver transplant evaluation.

- **Vegetation:** check for endocarditis keeping in mind that TEE is more accurate & may be performed after TTE for high suspicion.
- **Intracardiac thrombus**: mostly in a fib/flutter, CHF & post-infarction.
- **Aortic root dilatation**: usually is from HTN (normal <3. 8cm), ARBs are good HTN meds in this case (good data that protect aortic root)
- **Evaluation of prosthetic valve pathology**: check the gradients/regurgitation/vegetation.

In the case of stenosis, you should assess the gradients, valve area, & velocity through the valve, which, along w/ other criteria, is needed to assess severity & indication for surgical intervention.

Other cardiac tests

- **Treadmill stress EKG**:
  Indications: dx CAD, evaluate if known CAD & change in clinical status, risk stratify s/pACS, evaluate exercise tolerance, or localize ischemia. Preferred when applicable as it can tell the exercise tolerance (better prognosis if result is good- usually > 7 METS if male & >6METS if female). NOT applicable when EKG is uninterpretable (abnormal baseline like in LBBB, LVH w/ baseline ST depression, or presence of pacemaker). Do NOT do stress testing if the pt is unstable such as in ACS, acute CHF, acute pulm embolism, etc. Most often it is done in case of moderate probability of CAD. Stress test is NOT useful in case of low or high pretest probability as if it is high→ LHC is better test because normal stress test will NOT exclude CAD due to high % of false negative, & if it is low→ abnormal stress test will NOT change the management (like proceeding w/ LHC) because of high % of false positive results.
- **Treadmill stress echo:** if EKG is uninterpretable.

- **Pharmacological stress echo:** using dopamine, often ordered when the pt canNOT exercise (due to amputation, balance or pain problems, COPD, etc.).
- **Nuclear stress test (exercise or pharmacological)**: indicated also for moderate CAD suspicion (old MI will show no nuclear material uptake which indicates scar tissue while uptake at rest but NOT w/ exercise may indicate coronary stenosis which may benefit from LHC & revascularization).
- **CT scan coronary (angiogram):** noninvasive, mainly for young pts w/ atypical chest pain Sx & low suspicion of CAD, gives the CA anatomy. Heart rate should be low (55-60/min, give β blocker prn). **Coronary artery Ca score (CACS)**: mainly for screening purposes & predicting future risk of having CAD/heart attack.
- **Left heart catheterization (LHC):** for acute coronary syndrome (ACS- NSEMI/STEMI), high probability for CAD (typical angina Sx w/ risk factors), abnormal stress testing, systolic dysfunction w/ unexplained cause (evaluate new onset CHF), certain arrhythmias like sustained monomorphic Vtach or polymorphic Vtach, or s/p cardiac arrest. Intervention for revascularization can be: balloon angioplasty, stents (bare metal- BMS or drug eluted- DES). Consider CABG for multi vessel disease.
- **Right heart catheterization (RHC):** to assess hemodynamics (like RV end diastolic pressure- RVEDP & cardiac output for CHF pts), assess shock pts (cardiogenic vs. other reasons), & evaluate pulm HTN/calculate pulm resistance (& response to therapy).
- **Implantable Cardioverter Defibrillator (ICD):** **indication**: Malignant arrhythmias like V tach or V fib (especially s/p cardiac arrest), CHF w/ EF <35% (mainly after ≥3 months of optimal medical therapy), & age expectancy >1 year.

- **Pacemaker PM:** temporary at the bedside (for reversible causes) or permanent, for advanced AV blocks (Mobitz typeII or 3rd degree block). **Indication:** Symptomatic bradycardia w/ any AV block, Sick Sinus Syndrome (when you see sinus pauses on telemetry &/or escape rhythms like junctional rhythm → sinus dysfunction), tachy-brady syndrome (like in a fib with RVR → bradycardia when AV blocking agents are given), etc. Correlation of symptoms like dizziness & lightheadedness with the brady arrhythmias are supporting the need for PPM.

> **Attention:** Infx (or sepsis) can cause AV block → place temporary or temporary-permanent pacemaker prn until infx is treated & reassess (delay permenant PM so does NOT get infected).

- **EP studies:** new diagnostic/therapeutic studies for arrhythmias w/ ability to ablate abnormal pathways & arrhythmic foci w/ relatively high success rates (almost >95% for a flutter & >90% for a fib). Hold starting anti-arrhythmias meds (Amiodarone or Tikosyn) if your anticipating EP study as it will be hard to induce the arrhythmia in order to ablate it.

14. Hemoptysis

Expectoration of blood from lower respiratory tract; does NOT have to be accompanied by sputum production. Can range from blood-streaked sputum to massive expectoration & life-threatening bleeding. The amount of blood could be small but it is significant in the lungs (at that case, usually vitals are unstable w/ tachypnea, O_2 desaturation, & SOB).
If the source of expectorated blood is from upper respiratory tract/GI tract → pseudo hemoptysis. Massive hemoptysis: acute, life-threatening bleeding defined as ≥500 mL/24hr or bleeding rate ≥100 mL/hr.

Etiology

3B's → most common are bronchitis/PNA, bronchogenic CA, & bronchiectasis. Less common reasons: foreign body, airway trauma, Aspergilloma, CHF, Mitral Stenosis (MS), Pulm AVM, pulm embolism, TB, Wegener's Granulomatosis, good-pasture disease, coagulopathy: thrombocytopenia or anticoagx meds, complication of bronchoscopy or lung bx, & Cocaine (more of nasal bleeding from sniffing).

H & P

- Make sure it is a true hemoptysis, NOT just nasal or hematemesis
- Assess quantity, frequency, onset (acute or chronic), & presence of sputum
- Associated w/ SOB, fever, chills, & /or night sweats (infectious?)
- Diastolic heart murmur (for MS)
- Epistaxis, telangiectasias, renal insufficiency (for AVM & autoimmune etiology)
- Weight loss, cachexia, & smoker (malignancy)
- ASA, NSAIDS, & anticoagx

Tests:
- Pulse Ox, ABG, CXR
- CBC w/ diff, renal panel, UA
- Coagx status: PT/INR/PTT
- Sputum w/ gram stain & culture; acid fast stain, cytology
- ANA, ANCA, anti-GBM antibody
- BNP, TTE, high resolution CT
- Assess need for bronchoscopy w/ biopsy

Management

Massive hemoptysis
- Establish airway; if in respiratory distress, INTUBATE
- Transfuse blood products as needed: FFP, platelets, & pure RBC
- Bronchoscopy: balloon tamponade, iced saline lavage, topical vasoconstrictives (i.e. Epinephrine or topical thrombin), cautery, cryotherapy
- Angiography, embolization, & surgery

Stable hemoptysis
- Bed rest, supportive care w/ IV fluids, supplemental O_2, & serial CBCs. Treat underlying etiology. If you know the location of bleeding, make the pt turn toward the good lung to improve blood circulation & oxygenation.

Gastroenterology

15. Abdominal Pain

Abdominal pain is Sx that the vast majority of people will experience sometime in their life, & it has multiple causes.

History
- **Rule out the presence of the surgical abdomen** as this can kill the pt quickly. Make sure that the pt is hemodynamically stable.
- **Timing:** acute vs. chronic; gradual vs. sudden
- **Location**: localized vs. referred pain
- **Quality**: sharp, dull, tearing, burning, & boring; has the quality changed over time?
- **Prior episodes** of similar pain, relationship to **menstrual** cycles (female)
- **Associated Sx**: N/V, diarrhea, constipation, fever, etc.
- **Previous intra-abdominal procedures** such as appendectomy, cholecystectomy, & laparoscopies. Be concerned for small bowel obstruction secondary to adhesions.
- **Last bowel movement:** time & quality (soft or hard), this important as constipation can cause abdominal pain.

> **Attention:** flatulence is reassuring! (r/o complete Small Bowel Obstruction SBO)

- **Exacerbating or relieving** factors such as food, bowel movements, & deep breathe, positional, etc.
- **Presence of fresh blood** (hematochezia) vs. old blood (melena)

Physical exam
- Assess for any signs of an inferior MI as angina may present as epigastric pain
- Check for localized tenderness, rebound, guarding, & bowel sounds

- Stool guaiac PRN (but no need to perform FOBT if pt has frank blood because you already have your answer)
- Any woman of child bearing age who complains of lower abdominal/pelvic pain should get a pelvic examination
- **Murphy's sign:** pain on palpation of the right subcostal area during inspiration/p**cholecystitis**
- **Psoas or obturator sign:** pain upon passive extension of the thigh w/ knees extended while the pt is lying on their side → **appendicitis.**
- Rectal exam (should NOT be performed on neutropenic pts)
- **Carnett test:** used to distinguish intra-abdominal pain from abdominal wall pain. Press in the location of the pain & have the pt do a sit-up. If the pain worsens w/ the sit-up→ the pain is from the abdominal wall
- Pain that is out of proportion to the abdominal exam is suggestive of acute **mesenteric ischemia** (usually PMHx of CVA, CAD, PAD, or erectile dysfunction ED).
- Immunosuppressed pts may have benign exam despite a surgical abdomen.

Labs
- CBC, chemistry panel, liver function tests, amylase & lipase, lactate, Coagx panel
- Type & cross (if surgical abdomen or blood in stool)
- Urinalysis & urine pregnancy test
- In a pt w/ ascites that is having new abdominal pain or fever- a paracentesis must be performed to r/o SBP (spontaneous bacterial peritonitis). SBP is present if neutrophil count in the fluid is >250.

Abdominal pain: differential by pain location

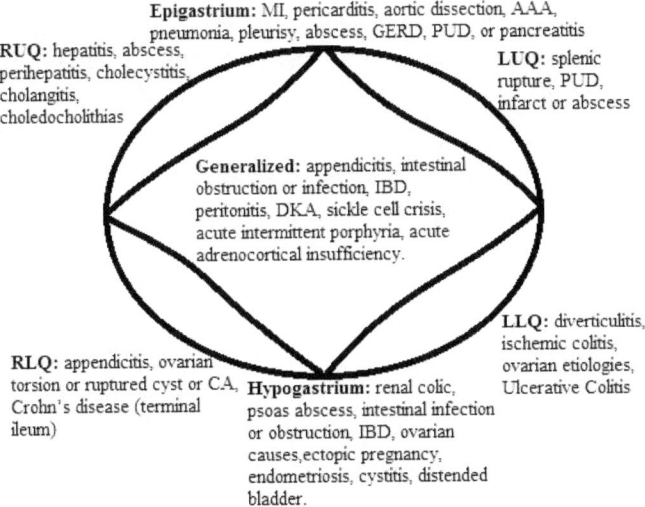

Epigastrium: MI, pericarditis, aortic dissection, AAA, pneumonia, pleurisy, abscess, GERD, PUD, or pancreatitis

RUQ: hepatitis, abscess, perihepatitis, cholecystitis, cholangitis, choledocholithias

LUQ: splenic rupture, PUD, infarct or abscess

Generalized: appendicitis, intestinal obstruction or infection, IBD, peritonitis, DKA, sickle cell crisis, acute intermittent porphyria, acute adrenocortical insufficiency.

LLQ: diverticulitis, ischemic colitis, ovarian etiologies, Ulcerative Colitis

RLQ: appendicitis, ovarian torsion or ruptured cyst or CA, Crohn's disease (terminal ileum)

Hypogastrium: renal colic, psoas abscess, intestinal infection or obstruction, IBD, ovarian causes, ectopic pregnancy, endometriosis, cystitis, distended bladder.

Radiology
- **Abdominal series:** r/o the presence of free air under the diaphragm, obstruction, volvulus, sentinel loop, toxic megacolon (> 7 cm in mid-transverse colon diameter), pleural effusion (pleurisy, pancreatitis if effusion is left-sided), etc.
- **Ultrasound:** to investigate hepatobiliary pathology if RUQ pain
- **CT abdomen/pelvis:** to r/o diverticular disease, appendicitis, & colitis
- Other studies will depend on the pt's specific situation

Management
- **If there is potential for a surgical abdomen, request a surgical consultation** & keep the pt NPO. Consider IV hydration. Type & cross for packed RBCs. Watch for septic/hypovolemic

shock. Hang appropriate abx (like Ciprofloxacin & flagyl for GI infx source) early if there is suspicion for ascending cholangitis, diverticulitis, sepsis, etc.

- Try a **GI cocktail (**30 ml of Mylanta or Maalox + 10 ml of viscous lidocaine ± 10 ml of Donnatal) if dyspepsia is a possibility
- **Consider starting a PPI drip** if pt w/ active GI bleed, & consult GI along w/ getting Hgb & hematocrit (H & H) Q6hr
- **Partial SBO** (usually from previous surgery adhesions) is managed conservatively by bowel rest w/ NG tube, IV fluid & pain management.

16. Nausea & vomiting (N/V)

Very common Sx. There is a vast majority of causes such as meds, chemo, underlying illness, reflux, etc. Always evaluate the pt at the bedside for new-onset vomiting or abdominal pain, persistent vomiting, or hematemesis. For symptomatic control, you can give the pt an antiemetic from the list below.

Medication

- **Ondansetron (Zofran):** serotonin 5-HT3 receptor antagonist. Very commonly used for any N/V w/ minimum side effect (prolong QT). Specific for cancer pts (chemo/radiotherapy) & surgery (prevent & Tx N/V).
- **Prochlorperazine (**Compazine) PO/IV/IM. Selectively antagonizes dopamine D2 receptors. **Side effects** include urinary retention, HoTN, spastic torticollis, dystonia (treat w/ Benadryl or Benztropine), cytopenias, & QT prolongation
- **Metoclopramide (**Reglan) PO/IV. Antagonizes central & peripheral dopamine receptors. **Side effects** include extrapyramidal Sx, urinary frequency, cytopenias, SVT, HTN, & sedation
- **Promethazine (**Phenergan) PO/IM/PR (antihistamine→hwill also produce sedation). Antagonizes central & peripheral H1 receptors (non-selective antihistamine). **Side effects** include sedation, cytopenias, & urinary retention
- **Lorazepam (**Ativan) IV/PO. Binds to benzodiazepine receptors, enhances GABA effects. NOT commonly used to Tx N/V alone but can be considered if sedation is needed as well. **Side effects** include delirium in the elderly & sedation.
- **Chemotherapy-induced:** Consider using serotonin antagonists, such as **ondansetron (Zofran)** or, as a last resort, **Marinol** (Cannabis derivative, very expensive, & appetite stimulator),

which works on cannabinoid receptors in the brain & is a schedule III drug. It is approved for chemotherapy-induced N/V.

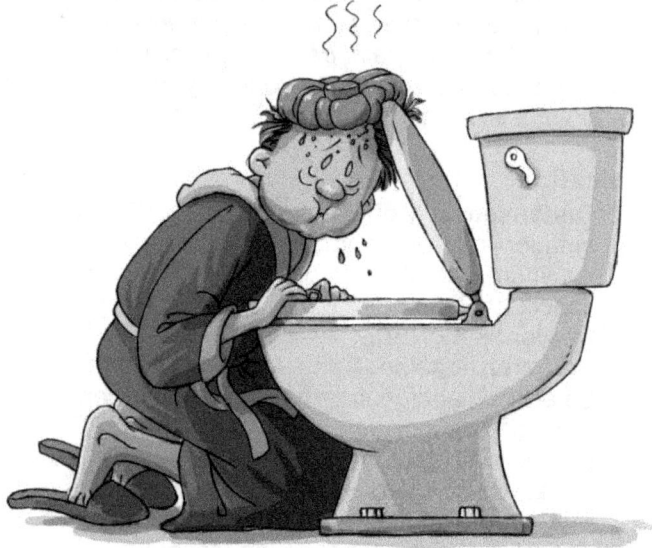

Nausea & vomiting are nonspecific Sx & can be very debilitating.

Special considerations

- **Fluid hydration:** If the pt canNOT tolerate PO, consider making the pt NPO & starting IV hydration along w/ PO/IV antiemetics (it is a reason for admission if N/V is refractory to PO antiemetics).

> **Attention**: Always ensure that the pt is hydrated & electrolytes are corrected.

- **Zofran has no sedating effect** (NOT dopamine antagonist) like Phenergan (1st generation antihistamine w/ antidopaminergic effect) &

Raglan (antidopaminergic effect w/ ↑ GI motility & lower esophageal tone)

- **Radiology:** If obstruction is a possible etiology, order an abdominal series x-ray. If there is evidence of an obstruction or ileus, place an NG Tube to help decompress the stomach
- **Usually NJ tube is for refractory N/V** pts to decompress the stomach for any etiology (NOT just obstruction).
- **Resolution:** As the Sx resolve, slowly advance the diet from clear liquid to full liquid to soft mechanical to regular (as indicated).

17. GI bleed

Symptoms
- **Upper:** N/V, hematemesis, coffee ground emesis, epigastric pain, & melena (black tarry stool from digested blood).
- **Lower:** Diarrhea, tenesmus, bright red blood per rectum, hematochezia (note: bloody stool can also be seen in rapid upper GI bleeding, but usually vitals will NOT be stable).

Etiology/Tx

Upper GI bleed	1. Peptic ulcer	50%: NSAIDs intake is common, H. *pylori* & ↑ gastric PH. Tx: EGD for possible clip or cauterization as indicated along w/ IV PPI, such as esomeprazole for 72 hrs then switch to high dose PO PPI like omeprazole 40mg BID.
	2. Varices	10-30%: esophageal (or gastric) from portal HTN. Tx: EGD w/ banding, octreotide IV for 2-5 days & prophylactic abx if the pt has cirrhosis (either ceftriaxone IV or norfloxacin PO). Consider TIPS for refractory cases.

Upper GI bleed cont-	**3. Esophagitis, gastritis, & duodenitis**	25%: due to NSAIDs, ASA, GERD & other meds, such as bisphosphonates & doxycycline. Tx: d/c the offending agent (NSAID, ASA, etc) & start PPI or H2 antagonist.
	4. Mallory-Weiss tear	Located at the gastro-esophageal junction from retching & vomiting. Tx: usually self-limited, but consider EGD if bleeding continues.
Lower GI bleed	**1.Diverticulosis**	Very common. Tx: usually self-limited, but if NOT then consider colonoscopy (for epinephrine injection, banding, APC, cauterizing). Last resort is to consult IR for embolization or general surgery for resection of the bleeding segment.
	2. Malignancy	Usually it is occult blood (positive FOBT & iron deficiency anemia). Management: colonoscopy
	3. Colitis	IBD (UC>CD), infx, mesenteric ischemia. Tx: steroids, abx or surgery evaluation as indicated.

Lower GI bleed cont-	4.Angiodysplasia (AVM), hemorrhoids, & anal fissures:	Rectal exam is diagnostic sometimes. Tx: usually self-limited, otherwise consider colonoscopy for intervention (or consult IR for embolization or surgery for resection).

Management for both upper & lower bleeding

First step:
Assess blood loss by vitals (tachycardia at >10% volume loss, orthostatic HoTN at >20% loss, & shock at >30% loss).

Resuscitate by two large IV lines & bolus fluid (mostly normal saline) until vitals stabilize. Type & screen 2-8 units PRBC on hold to transfuse if Hgb<7, but that threshold may be higher if there are comorbidities like CAD. Check PT/PTT/INR & reverse them w/ FFP, vitamin K, or platelets (keep >50k).

Check for organ failure: including AMS, urine output, liver dysfunction, & SOB.

Consider ICU if the vitals do NOT normalize after 1-2 L of IV fluids or if the pt had organ failure (abnormal LFTs, high Cr, AMS, CHF, SOB, or ongoing bleeding).

For ongoing bleeding call GI for possible scope & intervention to stop the bleed. Consider general surgery evaluation for the unstable pt w/ ongoing bleeding for possible laparotomy & resection.

Second step
Ask about the use of the following: NSAIDs, ASA, anticoagulants, antiplatelet agents, alcohol abuse, previous GI bleed, liver disease, or coagulopathy.

Sx & signs: abdominal pain, hematemesis or "coffee ground" emesis, passing melena/tarry stool.

Examination: vital signs, rectal examination for stool

color (melena vs. hematochezia vs. brown), anal fissures or hemorrhoids, & guaiac testing.

> **Attention**: Significant abdominal tenderness accompanied by signs of peritoneal irritation (e.g. involuntary guarding) suggests perforation.

NG tube w/ lavage is informative & easy test to localize the bleeding (upper or lower) if the diagnosis is unknown or can also clean the stomach before EGD. If it is an active upper GI bleed there will be fresh blood; if recent bleed & some digestion of blood has occurred → it will be coffee grounds; if it is non-bloody bile, the source may be lower or the bleeding was missed.
Keep the pt NPO (advance diet to clear liquid after diagnosis & Tx as indicated). Assess the comorbidities (to know when to transfuse & triage the pt to ICU vs. floor).

Special considerations
- **GI bleeding is NOT painful by itself;** therefore, abdominal pain (especially w/ guarding) may indicate perforation (order erect abdominal x-ray or KUB looking for free air & consider a stat general surgery evaluation). Consider mesenteric ischemia for pain out of proportion to signs, & worse w/ eating. The bleeding may indicate necrosis (surgery evaluation for resection may be needed to prevent sepsis).
- **Blood has a bowel stimulant effect** & causes diarrhea, so constipated pts are unlikely to have GI bleed.
- **Upper GI bleed is 80% of the GI bleeding** (that is why an EGD/NG tube is maybe indicated if the source of bleeding is unknown). A high percentage of GI bleeds are self-limited & will stop

spontaneously, however you still need to evaluate & treat due to a high percentage of recurrence.

- **An NG tube is part of the initial management** but be aware that it is contraindicated for variceal bleeding, therefore a detailed hx about cirrhosis, variceal bleeds, & endoscopic intervention like clipping is essential.
- **For acute bleeding** (NOT just GI bleeds), Hgb level may be falsely normal in the 1st few hrs due to plasma shifting. Vital signs are reflective of blood volume status more than the Hgb number, especially in the 1st few hrs.
- **Transfuse RBC**, regardless of Hgb level, if vitals are unstable after attempted fluid resuscitation.
- **Obscure bleeding** accounts for approximately 5% of the bleeds: no cause is found by upper & lower endoscopy. Many etiologies may be present. Management: repeat EGD & colonoscopy w/ push to the duodenum & ileum, capsule swallow (repeat to high sensitivity), Tc99 scan, tagged RBC scan, & angiography.
- **Stop & /or reverse any anticoagx.** It may be resumed after the bleeding stops & appropriate intervention is performed. Sometimes you need to weigh the pros & cons depending on the reason of anticoagx.
- **PPI drip** (which is NOT the same as PO/IV PPI) is indicated for upper GI bleed & it need to be continued for 72 hrs after EGD only if ulcer is seen w/ active bleeding/oozing or an obvious vessel in the base of the ulcer (high % of rebleeding in this case).

18. Diarrhea

Defined as↑ stool frequency & /or fluidity. Infx, toxins & drugs are common causes. Pseudomembranous colitis (C. difficile infx), abx, or fecal impaction (rectal exam can be diagnostic & therapeutic) are common causes for in pt diarrhea. Most of the time there is no need to identify the cause, especially if there are no alarming findings. Alarming findings associated w/ diarrhea include fever, significant abdominal pain, old age, duration>7days, hospital source, dehydration & blood or pus in the stool). Most infectious diarrheal conditions (including viral) are self-limited to 24hrs & Tx is Symptomatic (hydration is essential).

H & P

Ask about stool frequency, duration, blood or pus, N/V, abdominal pain, bowel sounds, fever, travel, diet & recent abx use. Assess hydration status (tachycardia, HoTN, orthostatic changes, skin turgor, capillary refill, urine output & mental status). If the episode of diarrhea is <24h w/ no comorbidities or other alarming signs like fever/abdominal pain/severe N/V, no need for further work up as a viral infx (which is self-limited usually lasting2-3days) is likely the cause & hydration will be sufficient.

Management:

- **Labs:** stool tests (WBC, fecal lactoferrin, fecal fat, C. *difficile* assay, FOBT, osmotic gap)
- **Early volume repletion**: to prevent dehydration (PO fluid, Gatorade, or IV NS depending on severity & comorbidities)
- **Abx**: for severe Sx while awaiting culture results like Ciprofloxacin/Norfloxacin, Bactrim, Metronidazole. Antidiarrheal meds can be used for non infx diarrhea (Loperamide, opiates, or Lomotil)

Special considerations

- **Diarrhea lasting>4 weeks is chronic.** If watery consider etiologies like **lactose intolerance:** diarrhea that ↓ w/ fasting/↑ osmatic gap/fecal tests negative for fat, WBC & blood). **Inflammatory** causes include: IBD, infectious, or ischemic & fatty diarrhea (e.g. chronic pancreatitis). Osmatic gap, 72 hr fecal fat, lactic acid, stool leukocytes & blood help to differentiate these inflammatory causes. .
- **Stool ova & parasites** should be ordered for pts w/ a hx of recent travel, exposure to outbreaks, or who are HIV positive
- **Metronidazole PO is 1st line abx against C. diff** & can be repeated if the pt fails to respond after a 1st course. IV Metronidazole is used in more severe cases (and if PO in NOT tolerated). Vanc PO is more expensive & can be considered as a 2nd line if metronidazole fail (differentiate between fail vs recerrence).

> **Attention**: unlike IV Metronidazole, IV vanc does NOT Tx c diff.

- **Severe comorbidities** (like CAD/arrhythmias/DM), old age & severe N/V unable to tolerate PO should be admitted to the hospital to insure appropriate IV hydration & electrolyte balance. PO hydration should be advanced as tolerated.
- **IBS** is a common cause & should be considered in cases of chronic diarrhea. Use the Rome criteria for diagnosis. Pts get relief after bowel movements.
- **Consider toxic megacolon** for IBD & immunocompromised pts due to ↑ risk of perforation. KUB & CT scan can be diagnostic. Tx: abx & steroids IV.

- **Symptoms that should prompt further work up** includes: Severe abdominal or rectal pain, Blood or pus in stool, black/tarry stools, fever, chronic diarrhea, weight loss, signs of dehydration (such as ↓d urination, lethargy or listlessness, extreme thirst, & a dry mouth). These diarrhea symptoms can be warning signs of conditions such as infection, irritable bowel disease, or pancreatitis, etc & needs more than symptomatic management.
- **Antimotility agents (like lomotil) are NOT indicated for infectious diarrhea** (treat the etiology & monitor improvement), except for refractory cases with abx.

19. Constipation

This is an important cause of abdominal pain. The vast majority of cases have no known etiology, but look for the obvious causes when working on a differential, such as dehydration, CCB, opioid use, hypothyroidism, anticholinergic meds, iron supplementation, & gastroparesis (from DM). Make sure there is no impaction or obstruction before starting medical therapy by doing a rectal exam & KUB. Always start from below first, if the pt agrees (like trying water enemas or rectal exam for stool impaction relief).

Management

- **Diet:** ↑ both total fiber & water intake. Psyllium 1 tsp daily-TID is a common 1st choice. If the pt is bed-bound & /or NOT drinking sufficient water, fiber can make the constipation worse.
- **Laxatives:** separated into 4 groups according to their mechanism of action
- **Emollients** (stool softeners): Mineral oil & docusate salts (Colace). Note: Mineral oil causes lipoid PNA if aspirated & ↓ the absorption of fat-soluble vitamins if given w/ meals.
- **Hyperosmolar agents**: Polyethylene glycol (MiraLax), lactulose, sorbitol, & glycerol. Note: Both lactulose & sorbitol are very effective & are highly recommended to use in chronic constipation if fiber & fluid supplementation alone do NOT work. Golytely is a similar laxative with some electrolytes which is indicated for bowel cleaning prior to colonoscopy
- **Saline laxatives:** Mg hydroxide (mild of magnesia) & Mg citrate (do NOT use w/ renal insufficiency because of Mg toxicity). This is usually NOT a good long-term option in the elderly.
- **Stimulant laxatives:** Castor oil, Senna (Senokot), & bisacodyl (Dulcolax). NOT recommended for long-term use. Dulcolax is a gastric irritant. Tablets

are enteric coated & should NOT be broken or chewed.

- **Prokinetics:** Reglan ↑ gut motility & is sometimes used in pts on opiates. However, do NOT give it if there is concern for obstruction, as this will make it worse. Erythromycine ↑ GI motility as well.
- **Opioid induced:** Methylnaltrexone (Relistor) is indicated for the Tx of opioid-induced constipation (OIC) in pts w/ advanced illness who are receiving palliative care when response to laxative therapy has NOT been sufficient. This is given in SQ form 8-12 mg Q daily & should be renally dosed. Naloxegol is another option.
- **Enemas:** can be used episodically for "salvage" therapy if an alternative bowel program has NOT produced a BM.

> **Attention:** Do NOT use Fleet's enemas in pts w/ renal insufficiency because of retention of phosphate (Naloxegol is another option).

- **Suppositories:** Both glycerin & bisacodyl (Dulcolax) can be used; however, they can be associated w/ cramping. They can also be used for "salvage" therapy.

Infectious Disease

20. Antibiotics (abx)

The best abx choice is to send a good culture specimen for sensitivity & choose the PO form (or the IV form at first & then switch to PO as indicated) w/ consideration of the side effect, expense, frequency, & comorbidity. You can follow up the infx resolution & the abx effectiveness by monitoring the fever, Sx, ESR/CPR, WBC & clinical improvement. Know what you are treating.

Common used abx

- **Vancomycin**: 1st line G + broad coverage, good for MRSA. IV form for broad coverage especially for sepsis or confirmed gram+ infx like strep & staph including MRSA. PO form is only for c diff infx as it does NOT absorb in GI track. Follow up blood troughs (usually after the 3rd dose) & adjust dose accordingly (therapeutic 15-20mcg/ml). Dosing is mostly BID for normal kidney but should be changed to either daily or q48hrs for AKI or CKD stage ≥ III (pharmacy can help dosing). On dialysis, give the dose after the session & get trough before it as 30% will be dialyzed out. Common empiric therapy w/ Zosyn.
- **Clindamycin:** gram + & anaerobic, PO for anaerobic infx mainly above the diaphragm like abscess, mild cellulitis out pt, aspiration PNA. Effective against community MRSA (althoughdoxycline & bactrim is better). Weak against group B strep & ↑risk of c. diff.
- **Daptomycin**: IV, Gram positive. Usually is NOT the 1st choice & is used when Vanc fails as it has great MRSA coverage. Do NOT use for respiratory infx (due to pulmonary surfactant inhibition effect on Daptomycin, but it is good for osteomyelitis & skin infx). Is NOT aminoglycoside.
- **Zosyn (Pipercellin/Tazobactam):** IV form, 1st line broad-spectrum coverage (Gram+, - & anerobic), for moderate & severe infx like nosocomial PNA,

106

abdomen infx (diverticulitis, abscess & peritonitis), skin infx. Does NOT cover MRSA. Can be used w/ Amikacin (aminoglycoside) to cover nosocomial pseudomonas. Common combination w/ Vanc as empiric Tx.

Same group: Unasyn (Ampicillin/Sulbactam), which is good against G- in general (Unlike Zosyn; it does NOT cover Pseudomonase). Augmentin (Amoxicillin/Clavulanate) is PO & common for out-pt mild-moderate infx like bacterial pharyngitis & sinusitis, animal bites, mild cellulitis (including diabetic foot), lower respiratory infx, & pyelonephritis.

- **Rocephin (Ceftriaxone):** IV cephalosporin, 3rd G, broad coverage (G+ & -), weak against Pseudomonas & anaerobic (do NOT use). Does NOT cover enteroccus (All cephalosporins do NOT cover it) or MRSA. Used for meningitis (especially caused by S. Pneumonia or meningococcal), gonococcalinfx, & prophylactic after sexual assault, UTI, skin infx, pelvic inflammatory disease, bone infx, & CAP (in combination w/ azithromycin).

  Same Group: Ceftaroline: 5th G cephalosporin & covers all MRSA; even Vanc resistant. **Cefdinir & Cefixime:** PO 3rd G cephalosporins (good for out pt therapy)

- **Azithromycin (z pack):** common out pt PO abx for atypical PNA, bronchitis, & GPC. 5 tablets 250mg each in 4 days. 2tab 1st day & then once qdaily. Yellow greenish phlegm does NOT automatically mean z pack.

- **Keflex:** 1^{st}G cephalosporin, PO for G +. Treats bone infx, UTI, otitis media, Upper RTI, strep pharyngitis. Mainly for skin flora & surgery likes them for prophylaxis. Great for cellulitis strep infx (good for MSSA).

  Same group: Ancef & Duricef

- **Linozolid:** PO or IV, Gram + including MRSA & Enterococcus. No Gram- coverage. Usually is a

2nd line after Vanc, especially for vanc resistance enterococcus. **Treat:** CAP, HCAP & skin infx. Does NOT treat bacteremia (NOT bactericidal).

- **Ciprofloxacin:** great for G- & pseudomonas (NOT good for G+). Used also for gastroparesis (from long lasting diabetes, manifests as early satiety & N/V) to ↑ GI motility. Prolongs QT interval. Use for: UTI, GI infx, CAP. Usually orally but available IV. Same group: Moxifloxacin & Levofloxacine (respiratory quinolones), which are preferred for CAP (good for G+ compared to Ciprofloxacin).

- **Amphotericin B:** IV, for severe fungal infx, mainly for AIDS & neutropenia pt or any immunosuppressed pt w/ presumed fungal infx for empiric fungal coverage. Order fungal blood culture before initiation. Nephrotoxic, hydration before & while on the med. Monitor electrolytes & kidney function.

- **Fluconazole:** common anti-fungal po drug for either Tx of common fungal infx especially candida (like PO thrush, vaginal candidiasis is, & even more severe cases like cryptococcal meningitis in AIDS) or prophylactic for immunosuppressed pts like in BMT. High doses can treat fungemia. Diflucan 150mg one dose po is a common Tx for vaginal candidiasis w/ white cheesy discharge (Vaginal Miconazole is another option). **Nystatin** is good for Candida infx like vaginal w/ creamy discharge, PO w/ white painful lesions or thrush, & skin candida (or Tania) w/ white flaky red skin w/ itching (use w/ combination of steroid like **Betamethasone** for Symptomatic relief). **Clotrimazole** topical is also effective against candida & most of other topical fungal infx (including athlete foot). Same group: **Voriconazol** (good for mold like aspergillus as fluconazole does NOT cover mold) & **Itraconazol**: for presumed serious fungal infx (comes in PO form).

- **Acyclovir:** effective against shingles if administered in 72 hrs from the blistering to reduce pain & ↓ duration. Another indication: herpetic encephalitis & genital herpes. Hydrate well before & during Tx due to risk of AKI. Same group: **ganciclovir** (mainly for CMV infx)

- **Metronidazole (Flagyl):** anerobic, 1st choice for clostridium difficile infx, vaginal infx (vaginosis w/ thin fishy smelling discharge & trichomoniasis w/ greenish yellowish discharge), Colorecatal infx, Giardia & Amebia infx. Category B in pregnancy (A accepted, D life threatening). Avoid Alcohol & educate about metallic taste. Mainly covers below the diaphragm.

- **Amikacin:** Aminoglycoside IV covers G- mainly. Treat: UTI, meningitis (G- infx), HCAP including Pseudomonas respiratory infx. Have nephro, neuro, & ototoxicity side effects.
  Same group: Gentamycin & **Tobramycin** (the best for pseudomonas & G-)

- **Doripenem:** broad coverage (GPC, GNB, & anerobic) except MRSA. From carbapenem group. Good for pseudomonas (intubation associated PNA or VAP). Only IV & is NOT usually 1st line Tx. Usually switched to it from zosyn if it fails for possible resistance (great gram negative coverage). At the same group: **Meropenem** which↑ risk of seizure in pt w/ CNS problem & **Ertapenem**, which is NOT covering pseudomonas but still good broad coverage (used once daily IV).

- **Aztreonam (monobactam abx):** IV/IM broad coverage for G- including pseudomonas aeruginosa (NOT good for G+ or anerobic). It is a synthetic monocyclic beta-lactam antibiotic (a monobactam). It is usually NOT the first line & used when other agents fail covering G- infx (like for UTI). Good option for penicillin allergy (cross reactivity is very low)

- **Bactrim:** Sulfa drug, usually PO. Very common use: PCP infx (& prophylactically) in immunosuppressed pts, UTI (lower for 3 days & upper use IV or PO for longer time, around

14days), skin (& soft tissue infx), CA-MRSA, & COPD exacerbation. Caution w/ sulfa allergy & in pregnancy (category C).

Special considerations:

- **Good culture specimens**
  - **Sputum:** Squamous epithelial cells line the mouth. If> 10 of these cells are present in the specimen then it is may be sputum w/ saliva but if<10 per hpf & >25 PMNs in the specimen, it is more likely to be from the lungs. Consider bronchoscopy by pulm for good sputum samples, if needed.
  - **Urine:** mid-stream clean catch (foley cath is NOT a good sample as it is may be colonized w/ bacteria).
  - **Abscess:** the wall of the cavity & NOT the pus (which is WBC & debris & may NOT have bacteria growing).
  - **Osteomyelitis:** Cx curettage from the ulcer base following superficial debridement of necrotic tissue. Organisms cultured from superficial swabs are NOT reliable for predicting the pathogens responsible for deeper infx. Bone biopsy & Cx is important before Abx (especially in chronic osteo)

> **Attention:** Findings that indicate abx are failing (need to switch abx for possible resistance) → persistent fever after 48-72 hrs, clinical deterioration, worsening erythema (like for cellulitis if it's pen marked)

- **MRSA abx:** Vancomycin, Daptomycin, Ceftaroline & Linezolid (for hospital acquired MRSA) & Doxcycyline, Bactrim, Rifampin & Clinamycin (for community acquired MRSA).

Pseudomonas abx: Zosyn, cipro/Levofloxacin, Cefepime, Ceftazidime, Mero/Imi/Doripenem (Ertapenem is NOT good for Pseudomonas), Topramycin/Gyntamycin/Amikacine, Aztreonam, Fasfamycin, & Colistin

- **Same bioavailability if they are given IV or PO:** Azithromycin, Levofloxacin, Ciprofloxacin, doxycycline, clindamycin, linezolid, & fluconazole.
- **You can choose either IV or PO abx** depending on the specific infx you are treating. Endocarditis may need IV abx for 6 weeks (PICC line will be useful) but treating something like PNA or UTI→ it's ok to start IV & switch to PO or even begin w/ PO. PO intolerance makes IV rout a good option. For bacteremia start IV & check for one negative blood Cx. After 2-3 days switch to PO if negative.
- **Antimicrobial stewardship program** (program for wise abx use) De-escalation of therapy, IV to PO conversions, Dose optimization, Guidelines & clinical pathways, Education (Colonization vs. infx). Implementation of an antimicrobial stewardship program helps: Improve pt outcomes, Improve pt safety, Reduces resistance, & Reduces cost

21. Fever

A normal temperature is 37°C & variation of +/- 1 degree is normal (low grade fever is 37. 5-38.0). Medically significant fever is >38 (or 100. 4 F).

H & P

Infected person exposure, chills, sweating, fatigue, rash, dehydration, or ↓ appetite. The degree of fever does NOT necessarily reflect the severity of the infx. Although infx is the most common reason for fever, consider other reasons such as cancer, infarction, CNS disease (e.g. hemorrhage), recent procedures (e.g. bronchoscopy), & meds.

Management

- **Tests:** CBC w/ differential (elevated WBC, & bandemia/left shift indicated infx), ESR & CRP, urine analysis, CXR, pan-culture (urine, blood & sputum) as indicated.
- **Tx:** Empiric abx (e.g. Vanc & Zosyn) can be started on pts w/ comorbidities (e.g. ESRD, CHF, COPD, cancer, etc.) after sending the cultures. You can stop abx if there are no indications of infx from the tests, or resume them if the source of infx found (de-escalate the abx depending on the sensitivity results). Consider meningitis & infective endocarditis (especially in pts w/ prosthetic valves) because these are catastrophic to miss.

Special considerations

- Elderly pts, pts w/ chronic hepatic or renal failure, & pts taking glucocorticoids may have **infx w/o fever.** A low temperature may be an indication of infx in these pt groups.
- Although subjective fevers need to be considered, **use objective measurements** for accurate assessment.

- **Check the absolute neutrophil count** because neutropenic fever is an emergency (start abx after sending pan-cultures, order a CXR & urine analysis as indicated).
- **Rash** (or skin erythema/abnormality) should be looked for in febrile pts. May indicate broad differential including viral infx (like Reckettsia), bacterial (like meningococcal infx), Lyme disease (tick bite), Mononucleosis (EBV) & cellulitis/osteomyelitis (NOT typically rash but erythema) & others.
- **Antipyretics** (acetaminophen & NSAIDs) can be given for fever. They do NOT cause harm & do NOT slow the resolution of common viral & bacterial infx. However, w/ bacterial infx, w/ holding antipyretic therapy can be helpful in evaluating the effectiveness of a particular abx, particularly in the absence of positive cultures of the infecting organism. Cold compressors can reduce fever as well.
- **Consider quick tests** like the Streptococcus test & influenza A/B swab as indicated to start abx or Tamiflu, respectively (effective in the first 1-2 days of signs & Sx).

> **Attention:** Do NOT culture more than once w/ in 24 hrs for pts who spike fevers (in case of an unidentified source of infx).

- **Reassess every day** whether the abx are still indicated & whether the fever is still present or not. Consider adding antifungal or antiviral meds for immunocompromised pts who are still febrile on empiric antibacterial coverage.
- **Postoperative fever** is common & etiology could be: atelectasia in 1-2 days postop (use incentive spirometry), HCAP in 1-2 days, Foley associated UTI in 3 days, cath related blood stream infx,

wonderdrug, surgical site infx in 5 days, DVT in ≥ 7days, or simply normal from the inflammation/stress of the surgery (or 5Ws: wind, water, wonderdrug, wound, walk)

22. White blood count

Quick facts regarding interpretation of WBC results, which are encountered every day in an in pt setting:

- **Elevated WBC count** (normal 4. 5-10k) is usually an indication of infx, especially if there are bands in the differential. Normal b & percentage is 3-5%, & bands>8% indicates infx. Bands reflect a "left shift" which is an ↑ in the number of immature leukocytes due to body's effort to make more WBCs rapidly.
- **Immune status should be assessed** for every pt, as the infx may present differently for immunocompromised pts (cancer, chemotherapy, steroids, etc.) versus immunocompetent (fever can be the only presenting Sx). Erythema/swelling for localized infx & elevated WBC may be absent due to the weak immune response. Abx coverage & prophylactic measures are different depending on the immune status as well.
- **Fever, sweat, fatigue, elevated ESR & CRP along w/ elevated WBC** are all indications for infx & immune response. The source of infx is important to identify (URI, UTI, abscess, PNA, meningitis, etc.), & the hx & physical can give clues to the source. In addition to the H & P, you can order pan-cultures w/ sensitivity (blood, urine, & sputum), UA, CXR, or lumbar puncture depending on the hx.
- **Neutrophil percentage is elevated mostly from a bacterial** infx (70% is normal), & lymphocytes from viral/fungal infx (20% is normal)
- **An elevated WBC is NOT always from infx:** although it is the most common reason. Steroid use, cancer, infarction, stress, recent procedure, anemia, burn, & pregnancy are also other causes of elevated WBC count that must be taken into account, especially if there are no other signs of infx.

- **A ↓ WBC count, <4K, can be a sign of infx as well,** especially in elderly pts, who no longer mount a good immune response.
- **Neutropenic fever** is an emergency. w/ this, the PO temperature is more than 38. 3°C & the absolute neutrophil count (ANC) is less than 500. Hospital admission & starting broad-spectrum IV abx are warranted, including possibly Vanc, Zosyn, & fluconazole. Most of the neutropenic pts w/ fever are cancer or post-chemotherapy pts.

> **Attention**: Neupogen (filgrastim) is a granulocyte colony stimulating factor, & can be used to ↑ WBC count post-chemotherapy if indicated. In most cases, it is used per Hem/Onc recommendations (no role in acute infx).

- **Often times, a very ↑ WBC count, >50K,** is assumed to be from leukemia/lymphoma, such as CML. However, a very ↑ WBC count can be caused by a leukemoid reaction from an infx & NOT malignancy.
- **Excessive IV fluids** can cause a dilution effect leading to a ↓ in all blood cell lines, including WBCs
- WBC count can be followed w/ a CBC on a daily basis to monitor the effectiveness of an abxTx. If it is still elevated after a day or two of initiating empiric abx, this may indicate a need to adjust abx.
- **Common WBC abnormal values:**
  1) **Spontaneous benign peritonitis** (SBP) WBC >250. Peritoneal dialysis PD fluid WBC >100 is indication of infx.
  2) **CSF** normal WBC 0-5, bacterial meningitis WBC>500, viral WBC>100
  3) **Arthrocentesis:** synovial fluid WBC>50K in bacterial septic joint while in crystal inflammation

(like gout) it can be up to 10-20K (synovial fluid smear & culture is needed)

4) **WBC>10 in urinalysis** is pyuria, one of the signs of UTI (normally <5 & absence of leukocyte esterase)

- **Elevated WBC (or ↓ <4K) is 1 out of 4 SIRS criteria.** SIRS can be diagnosed in the presence of 2 or more of the following (notice that HoTN is NOT part of SIRS criteria):
    1. ↑ temperature (>38. 3 or <36)
    2. Tachypnea (RR >20)
    5. Tachycardia (HR >90)
    6. WBC count >12K or <4K or >10% bands

23. Immune status

Immune-compromised pts need special attention because they do NOT have the ability to respond normally to an infx due to an impaired or weakened immune system. This inability to fight infx can be caused by a number of conditions including diseases (eg. diabetes, HIV, uremia), malnutrition, sickle cell disease, asplenia, chronic abx, elderly, ESRD on dialysis, cancer pts, & drugs (chronic steroids, transplant & autoimmune meds).

Assess immune status for all the pts, especially if their presenting illness is infectious (diagnoses & abx option are different depending on immune status).

> **Attention:** to unusual opportunistic infx like fungi (candida & cryptococcus), viruses (CMP, HSV & PK), & certain bacteria, which may NOT cause persistent infx in normal people. Signs of infx may NOT be as prominent in the immune-competent pts.

High-grade fever, elevated WBC w/ left shift, pain & guarding (in intra-abdominal infx), nuchal rigidity (in meningitis), & dysuria (in UTI) may NOT all be present in infx. High suspicion of infx & starting empiric abx coverage after sending the appropriate tests & cultures is very essential & may be life-saving.

> **Attention:** to non-specific findings like loss of appetite, fatigue, N/V, & HoTN (& other signs of shock). Consider infx.

Special considerations

- Most pts w/ immunodeficiency can safely receive all killed or inactivated **vaccines**. In contrast, live vaccines should NOT be given to pts w/ severe immune dysfunction.
- **Prophylactic abx** are indicated in pts w/ specific immunodeficiency disorders in order to prevent opportunistic infx: diclofenac for fungus, Bactrim for PCP infx (prophylactic dose every 48h), acyclovir.
- **PCP prophylaxis in non HIV pts:** Pts receiving a glucocorticoid dose equivalent to ≥20 mg of prednisone daily for one month or longer who also have another cause of immune-compromise; transplant pts (bone marrow or solid organs like kidney); pts receiving certain immunosuppressive drugs (purine analog or another T-cell depleting agent). Generally the need for prophylaxis is NOT permanent; however, it depends on the indication. HIV/AIDS pts w/ T4<200 may need Bactrim until their T4 ↑
- **Neutropenic fever:** a single PO temperature of >38. 3°C (101°F) or a temperature of >38. 0°C (100. 4°F) sustained for >1 hr (NOT just subjective fever) in pts w/ absolute neutrophil count (ANB) <500. There are many etiologies for neutropenia, but some of the most common are s/p chemotherapy & acute leukemia. Cover prophylactically w/ empiric parenteral abx therapy (such as vanc/zosyn), fluconazole, & acyclovir after sending pan cultures (blood/urine/sputum), & proceed w/ the work-up as indicated (CXR & urine analysis- UA). Neutropenic fever is a medical emergency & empiric antibacterial therapy should be started w/ in 60 minutes of presentation in all pts.

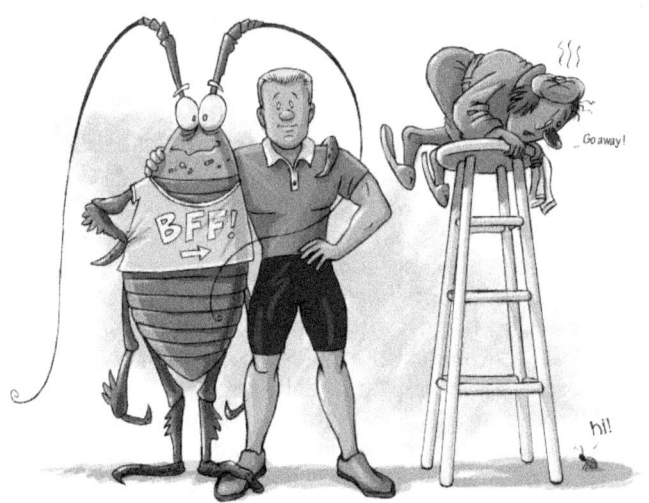

Immunocompromise pts manifest infx & get treated differently than immunocompetent.

24. Cellulitis & Osteomyelitis

Cellulitis

An infx of the skin & subcutaneous fat. Manifest as erythema (rubor), edema (tumor), warmth (calor), & pain (dolor) in the absence of underlying suppurative foci (such as an abscess which needs additional I & D). Lymphangitis (proximal red streaking) & regional lymphadenopathy may be present.

Predisposing factors include: disruption of skin barrier w/ trauma, as well as edema (venous insufficiency & CHF). Most commonly caused by beta-hemolytic Strep & Staph, including MRSA. Gram-negative bacilli are common in diabetic & immunocompromised pts Staph infx tend to be associated w/ abscess formation.

Management

Diagnosis is clinical & blood cx positive in few. Aspirate of bulla or pus from furuncle or pustule may provide diagnoses & culture sensitivity to narrow down the choice of abx. Mark the affected skin w/ a pen to monitor progression.

Tx

Abx include either **PO for mild cases** like Augmentin, clindamycin, or cephalexin or **IV if systemic toxicity** is present (empiric Tx w/ Vanc & Zosyn). Vanc is effective against MRSA. Doxycycline alone is also effective against MRSA & Strep for out pt. Re-evaluate the effected area & Teat the underlying predisposing conditions (like DM or lower extremities edema).

Special considerations

- **DDx:** necrotizing fasciitis (crepitus on physical exam & air on x-ray), gas gangrene (crepitus on exam), toxic shock syndrome, osteomyelitis, skin abscess (fluctuation & need surgical drainage), herpes zoster (vesicles in dermatomal distribution), DVT (mostly unilateral, warm, hx of immobility, especially after orthopedic procedures; Tx: anticoagx for 3-6 months if 1st time), venous insufficiency (bilateral, chronic, standing for long periods of time, no systemic Sx), crystal inflammation such as gout or pseudogout (mostly big toe joints, may show monosodium urate crystals from joint aspirate).
- **Necrotizing fasciitis** is a deep infx of the subcutaneous tissue that results in progressive destruction of fascia & fat. The affected area is usually erythematous (w/o sharp margins), swollen, warm, shiny, & exquisitely tender. There can be fulminant tissue destruction w/ systemic signs of toxicity, resulting in↑ mortality rates. Associated conditions include diabetes, substance abuse, obesity, immunosuppression, recent surgery, & traumatic wounds. Caused by either multibacteria or Group A Strep. **Tx:** aggressive surgical exploration & debridement of necrotic tissue, along w/ broad-spectrum empiric abx therapy & hemodynamic support.
- **Pts w/ lower extremities edema** may benefit from Tx w/ compressive stockings & diuretic therapy to prevent recurrent cellulitis.
- **Special cellulitis:** Cat bites (*P. multocida*); dog bites (*P. multocida, C. canimorsus*); penetrating injury like nails (*Pseudomonas*); gardening injury (*Sporothrix*).

> **Attention**: Skin flora like Strep & Staph are still the most common causes of the cellulitis after the bite injury (treated w/ Vanc for in pt & clindamycin or Bactrim for out pt). Vaccination status for tetanus & rabies should be explored.

- **IV abx** can be started for few days & then switched to PO if pt is improving.

Acute Osteomyelitis
Infx of bone due to hematogenous seeding (S. aureus) or direct spread from contiguous focus from skin damage from trauma (S. aureus & S. epidermidis). Local findings such as erythema, warmth, swelling, & pain may be present along w/ systemic signs such as fever, night sweats, & malaise.

Management:
Identification of the causative organism is key. Blood cultures & needle bx or surgical sampling. Radiologic work up: X-ray (needs time to be abnormal), MRI (detects early changes) & bone scan (↓ specificity as it will be positive in cellulitis as well). Tx: Abx (based on Cx data) for 4-6 weeks. WBC count, ESR & CRP are significantly elevated & they can be monitored if abx resistance is a concern. ID & orthopedic surgery may need to be consulted.

Chronic osteomyelitis
May NOT see leukocytosis. The key is to identify the causative organism (by a surgical biopsy/ culture before starting abx) & start abx according to C & S. Consider surgery evaluation for acute osteomyelitis that fails to respond to medical therapy, chronic osteomyelitis, complications of pyogenic vertebral osteomyelitis (e.g., early signs of cord compression, spinal instability,

epidural abscess), & infected prosthesis. Best evaluated by X-ray & MRI.

Diabetic foot: infected neuropathic foot ulcer. Usually is complicated w/ arterial impairment. Tx: bed rest, elevation, non–weight-bearing status, wound care, abx. For mild or out pt, use Augmentin or Cephalexin. Add Bactrim if MRSA is suspected. For severe or in pt: Vanc & (Zosyn or Imipenem) for 6 weeks.

25. Infective endocarditis

Infx of the endocardium manifested by the protypical lesion, vegetation, most commonly located on heart valves. Consider it in case of Bacteremia (mostly w/ gram + cocci as they "stick" to the heart valves unlike gram -bacillus), unknown fever source, new onset heart failure, acute weight loss & pts w/ risk factors like prosthetic valves (bio or mechanical).

Etiology
Typical organisms causing endocarditis are: Staphylococcus aureus (commonly associated w/ intravascular devices & injection drug abuse), Streptococci (group B & viridans group), HACEK group (Hemophilus, Actinobacillus, Cardiobacterium, Eikenella & Kingella). Prosthetic valve endocarditis is most often associated w/ S. aureus, coagulase negative staph, enterococci, gram-negative bacilli, viridans strep & Candida SP.

Types
Endocarditis is typically classified into *acute, subacute, & prosthetic valve endocarditis.* Acute endocarditis typically presents over 5 to 10 days & is often associated w/ Staphylococcus aureus & gram-negative bacilli (less common). Subacute endocarditis typically presents over weeks to months & is associated w/ Streptococcus species.

Clinical features
Fever, chills, sweats, anorexia, weight loss, malaise, myalgias & /or arthralgias, back pain, new or changing heart murmurs, splenomegaly, clubbing, Osler's nodes, Janeway lesions, subungual hemorrhages, Roth's spots, petechiae, neurologic manifestations.

125

Work-up

Positive blood cultures & demonstration of vegetations on an echocardiogram are two major criteria for diagnosis (see below for criteria). Other lab abnormalities which are seen in IE are anemia, leukocytosis, hematuria, elevated ESR, CRP, RF, ↓ serum complement.

Diagnosis

For clinical diagnosis, Duke Criteria are often used:

Major criteria	Minor criteria
Positive blood culture: Typical microorganism from 2 separate blood cultures, OR For atypical microorganisms, persistently positive blood cultures (blood cultures drawn 12 hrs apart or all of the 3 sets of blood cultures or majority of4 separate blood cultures are positive, w/ 1st & last culture drawn >1hr apart), OR Single positive blood culture of Coxiellaburnetii or phase I IgG antibody titer of >1: 800. **Evidence of endocardial involvement:** Positive echocardiogram:Oscillating intra-cardiac mass on valve or supporting structures, **OR** Abscess, **OR** New partial dehiscence of prosthetic valve, **OR** New valvular regurgitation.	1. **Predisposing heart condition of IV drug abuse.** 2. **Fever** (>38 degree Celsius). 3. **Vascular phenomena** (Arterial emboli, septic emboli, mycotic aneurysm, intracranial hemorrhage, conjunctival hemorrhage, Janeway lesions). 4. **Immunologic phenomena** (glomerulonephritis, Osler's nodes, Roth's spots, rheumatoid factor). 5. **Microbiologic evidence:** + blood culture but NOT meeting major criteria or serologic evidence of activeinfx w/ typical microorganism.

For diagnosis, 2 major OR 1 major & 3 minor OR 5 minor criteria are essential.

Please note

- TTE is accurate in only about 65% cases of endocarditis. Hence, if clinical suspicion is high, always order a TEE, which is accurate in >90% cases.
- When endocarditis is very likely, a negative TEE does NOT exclude diagnosis & should be repeated in 7-10 days.
- TEE is the optimal method for diagnosis of Prosthetic valve endocarditis or detection of myocardial abscess, valve perforation or intra-cardiac fistula.
- Follow-up TEE or TTE is needed to re-assess vegetations, complications, or Tx response.

Management

IV abx for extended periods of time (usually for 6 weeks, consider PICC line). Start w/ broad empiric Tx like Vanc & Zosyn (G+ coverage is essential) & then narrow down depends on susceptibility (usually ID are involved).

Endocarditis prophylaxis

1. Prophylaxis is recommended for the following conditions:
    a. Prosthetic valves.
    b. Previous endocarditis.
    c. Unrepaired congenital heart disease, including palliative shunts or conduits.
    d. Repaired congenital heart disease w/ prosthetic material during 1st 6 months of procedure
    e. Cardiac valvulopathy in transplant recipients.
2. Dental, PO or respiratory tract procedures require prophylaxis in the above-mentioned conditions.
3. GI & genitourinary procedures DO NOT require routine prophylaxis; however, high-risk pts infected or colonized w/ enterococci should receive

amoxicillin, ampicillin or Vanc prior to urinary tract manipulation.
4. Prophylaxis is recommended for procedures on infected skin, skin structures or musculoskeletal tissue for conditions mentioned above.
5. Prophylaxis is w/ amoxicillin or ampicillin 30 mins to 1 hr before procedure (clindamycin/cephalexin/azithromycin/clarithromycin/clindamycin if pt is penicillin allergic).

Special considerations
- In general, consider infective endocacarditis if you have sick pts with more than one damaged organs at the same time w/o good explanation like new onset CHF & AKI (from valvular disease from the vegetations & from septic embolism)
- Streptococcus gallolyticus (previously known as Streptococcus bovis) is associated w/ colon polyps & tumors.

> **Attention**: G- organisms bacteremia usually does NOT cause IE (no need for TEE unless you have very high suspicion) while G+ organisms does (sticky organisms).

- Unusual form of endocarditis resulting from endocardial damage due to abnormal blood flow is NBTE (non-bacterial thrombotic endocarditis); seen commonly in valvular abnormalities such as mitral & aortic regurgitation, ventricular septal defect & congenital heart defects. When uninfected vegetations occur in malignancy, chronic diseases, Systemic Lupus Erythematosus (SLE) & anti-phospholipid syndrome, it is known as marantic endocarditis.

26. Clostridium difficile infection (CDI)

C. difficile infx is a major cause of in pt gastrointestinal illness. C. difficile is a gram-positive, spore-forming, normal flora of the GI tract mostly spread by the fecal-PO route. Soap & water is the best for prophylaxis (alcohol foam does NOT eliminate spores).

Risk factors

Recent abx use is the main culprit, especially clindamycin, cephalosporins, & fluoroquinolones. Though, any abx can predispose to *C. difficile* overgrowth, including Vanc & metronidazole. Nursing home pts, elderly, immunosuppressed, & pts w/ altered GI anatomy (e.g., ileostomy, colostomy) are at ↑ risk.

Clinical features

Typical presentation is profuse watery diarrhea, lower abdominal pain/tenderness, & often extremely foul-smelling stool (nurses usually suspect that first).

Laboratory tests

The most accurate test is stool *C. difficile* antigen PCR. The disadvantage is that it takes around 24-48 hrs to return from the lab. Get CBC & CMP to assess severity.

Classification

Used to decide on Tx options, including possible ICU care.

- **Mild:** Diarrhea is the sole Sx.
- **Moderate:** Diarrhea plus additional signs & Sx NOT meeting criteria for severe or complicated CDI.
- **Severe:** Hypoalbuminemia (albumin <3), a WBC count >15 k, & abdominal tenderness. **Complicated CDI pts who need to be considered for ICU:** HoTN w/ or w/o vasopressors, fever > 38. 5°C, ileus, abdominal

distension, mental status changes, WBC count >35, 000or <2, 000, serum lactate level >2. 2 mmol/L, & any signs of end-organ failure.

Tx

Can be initiated before laboratory confirmation for pts w/ a ↑ pre-test suspicion. The offending abx should be stopped. If abx must be continued, treat w/ abx less known for causing CDI, such as aminoglycosides, macrolides, Vanc, or tetracycline.

- **For mild-to-moderate CDI**: PO metronidazole 500mg TID x10 days should be used. If the pt fails to respond to metronidazole therapy, a change in therapy to PO Vanc should be considered.
- **Severe or complicated disease:**
  w/o ileus → PO Vanc is administered (in addition to IV metronidazole)
  w/ ileus →Vanc delivered PO & per rectum plus IV metronidazole is to be given. Additionally, supportive care w/ fluid resuscitation, electrolyte replacement, & DVT prophylaxis should be continued. A CT abdomen & pelvis is recommended in pts w/ complicated CDI, as is a surgical consult due to possible need for subtotal colectomy & ileostomy, which is associated w/ ↓ mortality.
- **Recurrent disease:** The **first recurrence** of CDI should be treated w/ the same regimen used for the initial episode. However, if infx is severe, PO Vanc should be used. The **second recurrence** should be treated w/ Vanc PO. For a **third recurrence** after a pulsed Vanc regimen, fecal microbiota transplant (FMT) should be considered.

Special considerations

- **Fidaxomicin** was approved for mild-to-moderate CDI & was non-inferior to Vanc in phase III trials & **Fecal microbiol transplant (FMT)** has shown promising results in trials for recurrent CDI as mentioned above.

- **PO Vanc is expensive** but PO metronidazole is cheap.
- **Do NOT test C. diff in pts w/o diarrhea** (unless you have another reason like leukocytosis w/o known source). Monitor response to Tx by decreasing bowel movement numbers per day. Recovery is monitored clinically (usually no need to test negative C. diff as it can be positive after the Tx for months w/o the need to repeat abx & it is NOT a sign of Tx failure).
- **Start counting 14 days of anti C diff abx (like Flagyl or Vanc) from the time you stop the offending agent** (like Clindamycin). Do NOT undertreat in order to avoid recurrence.

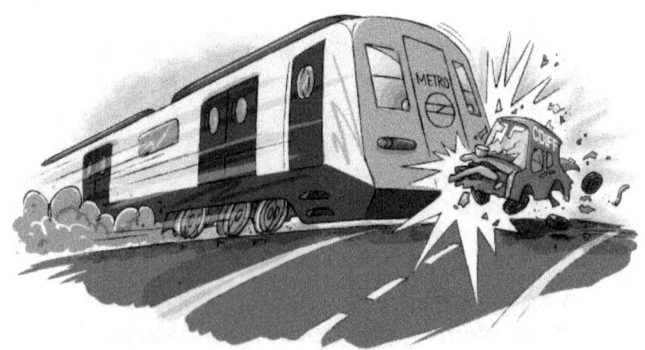

*METROnidazole is effective against **C diff** infx.*

27. Methicillin-Resistant Staphylococcus Aureus (MRSA)

Thisis a major cause of morbidity & mortality in hospitals. It can cause PNA, bacteremia & skin & skin structure infx (SSSIs). Tx has become challenging because of resistance & limited availability of antimicrobial agents. Moreover, there has been an emergence of community-acquired strains (CA-MRSA), which sometimes have a higher virulence than hospital-acquired ones.

Community-acquired MRSA

Clindamycin, trimethoprim-sulfamethoxazole (TMP-SMX) & tetracyclines (doxycycline) are recommended as first line agents for CA-MRSA, but should NOT be used for hospital-acquired strains due to ↑ resistance. Out of the 3 agents mentioned above, only clindamycin has good activity against both MRSA & beta-hemolytic Streptococci. Usually, in skin infx thought to be due to MRSA, empiric coverage for both MRSA & Streptococci is needed. However, using clindamycin as a sole agent can lead to resistance. Hence, TMP-SMX or doxycycline in combination w/ a beta-lactam agent, such as ampicillin or amoxicillin, is preferred.

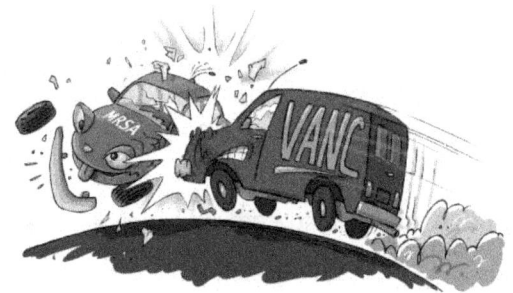

*VANcomycin is the 1ˢᵗ empiric IV Tx of choice for **MRSA**; especially for in pt.*

Hospital-acquired MRSA: Nursing homes, dialysis centers, or any long-term healthcare facility. Has been treated w/ IV **Vanc** for several years. It is cheap, effective, & has years of experience behind its use as a first line agent. However, in recent years, there have been reports of ↑ resistance & rising minimum inhibitory concentrations (MICs).

There are several reports of emergence of VRSA (Vanc resistant *S. aureus*), VISA (Vanc intermediate *S. aureus*), & HVRSA (heterogeneous Vanc resistant *S. aureus*). However, as of now, it is still used as a first line agent for MRSA.

Vanc is a bactericidal agent & acts by inhibiting cell wall synthesis. It is used only in IV formulation (unless specifically treating *C. difficile* infx), & requires dose adjustment in renal insufficiency. Nephrotoxicity & red man syndrome are among the most common adverse effects associated w/ it, & require stopping the drug. Trough (blood level) should be checked regularly to assure therapeutic levels (make sure it is a true trough by checking it just before the next dose or before HD).

Linezolid is another agent that can be used in both PO & IV formulations. It has good lung penetration & is recommended for MRSA PNA NOT responding well to Vanc & in pts being discharged back to a nursing home on PO meds.

Daptomycin is among the newer agents approved for Tx of MRSA. It is used for MRSA bacteremia, but is NOT recommended for use in MRSA PNA as it is inactivated by pulm surfactant. Additionally, it can be used for complicated skin infx & infective endocarditis. Adverse effects include myopathy (monitor CPK), peripheral neuropathy, & eosinophilic PNA.

Ceftaroline (Cephalosporins) is good for MRSA & is approved for PNA & cellulitis infx (NOT the 1st line though)

Nephrology

28. Acute kidney injury (AKI)/Chronic Kidney Disease (CKD)/End stage Renal Disease (ESRD)

AKI:
General: most common practical definition is an acute ↑ in serum Cr >0.3 from baseline (so it can occur in normal kidneys & impaired kidneys like CKD). Prerenal & postrenal causes should be distinguished from intrinsic renal parenchymal disease because they are rapidly reversible. Also divided into oliguric (<400 ml/24hr) & nonoliguric (>400 ml/24hr). The lower the urine output, the worse the prognosis.

Work up for AKI:

- Check **dehydration**, ↓ oral intake, HoTN (infx/sepsis in general) or bleeding as prerenal is very common cause for AKI & it is easy reversible by IV/PO fluid. Prevent expensive work up by good chart review & history.
- Check **new meds**, which maybe are NOT kidney friendly like ACEi/ NSAIDs & stop them/ monitor improvement (may NOT need further testing).
- **Urine analysis (UA)** to check for UTI, urine protein, blood, etc. Urine sediment examination for casts, cells & crystals are best done by Nephrology. The presence of WBC casts & Eosinophils in the urine may indicate Acute Interstitial Nephritis AIN (a type of intrinsic AKI usually caused by Beta-Lactam Abx). RBC casts are highly suggestive of glomerular pathology.
- **Kidney US** if you suspect postrenal (look for obstruction/hydronephrosis). Relief obstructions ASAP w/ either foley cath (if BPH) or nephrostomy (for maybe uretral stricture or

stones) depends on the level of the obstruction. Anuria or oliguria is maybe a clue (consider foley cath or bladder scan first before formal abdominalUS; cheaper/faster)

- **FeNa** can differentiate prerenal from intrinsic (like Acute Tubular necrosis ATN) AKI in pts w/ oliguria (although it is also commonly used w/ nonoliguric pts but has lower sensitivity). ↓ FeNa tells you that the kidney is "working" & keeping or reabsorbing most of the filtered Na to the blood, so the AKI can be treated w/ fluid because it is due to a prerenal etiology. If the pt is on diuretics, check FeUrea instead of FeNa (diuretics impair renal ability to reabsorb Na & give false values). FeNa can be calculated online by the values of both urine & serum Cr & Na.

> **Attention to** AKI from CHF exacerbation also could cause low FeNa but should NOT be given IVF

- Consider **peripheral blood smear** to check for schistocytes when there is suspicion for HUS, TTP, malignant HTN, or scleroderma renal crisis.
- **Look for signs of cirrhosis in pts w/ evidence of chronic liver disease or BNP/CXR in pts w/ CHF** as they both have ↓ effective intravascular volume perfusing the kidneys even though pts usually are volume overloaded. Cardiorenal & hepatorenal syndrome are hard to treat.

Management:
- **Start IV normal saline** for pts w/ volume depletion.
- **You can try albumin** for those w/ cirrhosis & intravascular volume depletion.

- **Review meds:** stop ACE inhibitor, diuretics, NSAIDs & any nephrotoxic meds
- **In case there is urinary obstruction:** place urinary cath to relieve bladder outlet obstruction. If the obstruction is above the bladder, consult urology for nephrostomy placement.
- **Monitor daily Cr & electrolytes** especially K, & daily ins/outs. Assess daily need for dialysis & signs of renal recovery.

CKD:

CKD is characterized by abnormality of kidney function (hematuria, proteinuria, etc) or an alternation in kidney function for > 3 months (elevated serum Cr & $\downarrow$ eGFR as above). Always compare Cr level to baseline values. Elevated Cr is a good indicator for impaired renal function but always calculate eGFR as it is takes into consideration other factors like: pt's age, sex & race. As Cr is a muscle product, $\downarrow$ body muscle mass (in thin pts) can give a falsely normal or low [Cr] even in the presence of CKD.

Stage	GFR
1*	≥90
2*	60–89
3a	45-59
3b	30-45
4	15–29 (needs preparation for kidney replacement therapy, dialysis)
5	<15 or on dialysis

*Need to have anatomical or functional renal abnormalities.

Attention: DM & HTN are common etiologies for CKD.

Common Etiologies:

- **Diabetic kidney disease:** Look for microalbuminuria, followed by proteinuria & declining GFR. The presence of retinopathy strongly suggests coexisting nephropathy.
- **Glomerular disease:** Look for glomerular hematuria, proteinuria, & HTN; if w/ systemic manifestations, lupus nephritis & postinfectious GN. If nephrotic syndrome is present look for FSGS, membranous nephropathy, minimal change disease & amyloidosis. Kidney biopsy is often needed to make the diagnosis.
- **Tubulointerstitial disease:** look for proteinuria, glycosuria, pyuria & leukocyte casts, as well as, papillary necrosis on ultrasound.
- **Structural disease**: like autosomal dominant polycystic kidney disease (ADPKD): HTN, hematuria & family hx of CKD.

Management:

- **Begin restriction** of Na (<2g/day if comorbid CHF or refractory HTN), Low K (60mEq/day), & low phosphorus (800-100mg/day) diet might be needed in patients with more advance CKD.
- **For HTN:** use ACE-I or ARBs, diuretics are commonly needed (use loop diuretics rather than thiazide for GFR<30)
- **For persistent microalbuminuria:** start ACE-I or ARBs even if pt is normotensive (for the kidney protection effect).
- **Anemia:** erythropoietin to maintain Hg between (10-11) & iron to maintain iron stores. Always check iron levels before stating erythropoietin as iron deficiency can coexist w/ anemia of chronic disease from CKD. Correct iron deficiency before starting erythropoietin.
- **Hypocalcaemia & Hyperphosphatemia:** Can lead to secondary hyperparathyroidism

manifested by & elevated Parathyroid hormone (PTH).

1. Low phosphorus diet.
2. **Correcting Hyperphosphatemia** – Use Ca based binders including: Ca Carbonate & Ca Acetate. Non-Ca based alternatives like Sevelamer

- **Metabolic acidosis:** Bicarb HCO3 therapy to maintain HCO3 between (20-26). Usually 650-1300mg TID.
- **Vitamin D deficiency:** CKD leads to ↓ production of calcitriol, which is the active form of Vit D. This also causes ↑ of PTH. Can give calcitriol once 25-OH Vit D repleted.

Special considerations:

- **Refer CKD to nephrologist in stage ≥3** for cause identification, complication management & timely preparation for transplant or dialysis (as AV fistula/graft needs weeks to months to maturate & be ready to be used). Avoid frequent BP measurements & unnecessary PICC/central line in such pts to save those peripheral & central veins for future possible HD life-saving accesses (consult nephrology in non-urgent cases for further recommendation)
- **Kidney transplant:** is associated w/ superior quality of life & is less expensive compared w/ long-term dialysis. All pts w/ ESRD are considered candidates for kidney transplant unless they have systemic malignancy, chronic infx, severe cardiovascular disease, or neuropsychiatric disorders. Transplantation is particularly beneficial in young pts.
- **Hemodialysis HD indication:** 1-refractory hyperkalemia (NOT responding to Kayexalate, insulin/dextrose, albuterol & lasix), acidemia (NOT responding to HCO3 PO or IV), or volume overload (NOT responding to lasix or other loop

diuretics). 2-Signs & Sx of uremia (AMS, asterixis, pericardial friction rub, vomiting).

- **ESRD pts on HD**: usually get 3 session of HD a week. Compliance w/ HD, fluid restriction & ↓ Na/K/phosphate diet should be assessed regularly & monitoring body weight (for fluid overload) can be very informative. Pulm edema/congestion/CHF exacerbation may occur very often in non-compliant pts which necessitates urgent HD.
- **FE (Na) interpretation in pts w/ oliguria:** If >1% consider tubular damage such as ATN. If <1% & UA is normal, consider prerenal azotemia
- **ACEi is expected to ↑ Cr** as it lowers the intraglomerular pressure from vasodilatation on both afferent & efferent arterioles but more on efferent arterioles. This ↑ is NOT considered an AKI unless it is > 30% from baseline (so repeat Cr 2 weeks after ACEi initiation). Stop ACEi in such case & any case of AKI to avoid further compromising of renal perfusion.
- **Adjust medication doses according to eGFR** to prevent toxicity, especially meds cleared renally. Meds stay in the system longer in the case of AKI/CKD. (e.g. cause AMS in case of morphines & benzos & bleeding in case of novel anticoagx).

29. Urinary tract infection (UTI)

Categorized, mostly, into either upper or lower UTI.

Lower UTI Sx: dysuria, ↑ frequency, urgency, hematuria & suprapubic pain while **upper UTI** (or pyelonephritis) **Sx:** fevers, chills, sweats, N/V, vomiting, diarrhea, & flank or abdominal pain. Lower UTI Sx may also precede these Sx.

Another way to categorize UTIs:
uncomplicated which is the 1st lower UTI for female or **complicated** which is the rest (like any upper UTI for either sex, any UTI in male, recurrent lower UTI in female).

Urine analysis (UA) is an easy, cheap & fast diagnostic test for UTI (although Sx & physical exam can be enough). Elevated WBC, esterase (sign of WBC), nitrates (sign of bacteria) & RBC (±) presence along w/ bacteria is positive in any UTI. Leukocytosis & bandemia along w/ positive blood culture can be found in upper UTI.

Management:
Uncomplicated UTI: You can start the empiric Tx based only on the Sx.
- **In non-pregnant female:** 3 days of TMP-SMX, 5 days of Nitrofurantoin or single dose (3 grams) of Fosfomycin
- **In pregnant female:** Ampicillin, Fosfomycin, Nitrofurantoin, Keflex, Aztreonam or Cefixime for 7-10 days (longer than usual). Repeat urine Cx to assure resolution in a monthly bases & Tx even asymptomatic bacteriuria in pregnancy as they are high risk for frank UTI (30-40%) due to progesterone effect as a smooth muscle relaxant.

Complicated UTI: Obtain urine culture then initiate Tx empirically for 7-14 days w/ Ciprofloxacin PO or IV (be aware of QT prolongation & get a baseline EKG, consider another abx if QT is already prolonged or pt is on other QT prolonging meds like haldol).

Upper UTI (pyelonephritis):
- **For young pts who can tolerate PO intake & are relatively healthy:** consider PO fluoroquinolone like Ciprofloxacin for 7 to 14 days (you may NOT need urine analysis or urine culture). Consider hospital admission & IV Ciprofloxacin if the pt has N/V & then discharge on PO Ciprofloxacin when PO is tolerated.
- **Choose broad-spectrum coverage w/ extended-spectrum beta lactam like zosyn or carbapenem in the following settings:** suspected resistant organism (like recurrent UTI & indwelling foley cath), recent abx use, urinary obstruction & immunosuppression. You can add gram positive coverage like Vanc in case of septic shock or complicated pts (like elderly w/ multiple comorbidities)
- **Obtain Renal Ultrasound or CT** for persistent fevers or continuing Sx after 72 hrs of abx to evaluate for complications of pyelonephrosis (e.g., perinephric abscess).
- **Obtain Urine culture** especially for hospitalized pts & de-escalate (optimize) abx if empiric agents like Zosyn/vanc were started

Special consideration:
- **Pts w/ chronic foley cath** may always have UA positive for WBC, esterase & bacteria which is due to colonization; so do NOT treat unless Sx are present (elevated blood WBC, fever, dysuria or any systemic infx signs).

> **Attention:** UTI is a common reason for AMS or GI Sx like N/V in elderly; so do NOT forget to check UA in elderly.

- **Treat asymptomatic bacteriuria** (positive bacteria in UA w/ no WBC or esterase) only in pregnant women & prior to invasive urologic procedure. Some pts w/ chronic indwelling Foley like spinal injury pt, or prostate cancer pts, as well as ESRD pts on HD can have positive UA (+ bacteria, nitrate & esterase) but Tx w/ abx is NOT indicated unless they are Symptomatic (fever, dysuria, elevated WBC, or sepsis). Usually the bacteria in this case are very resistant & strong abx like imipramine should be reserved for a later time when the pt is in real need (eg: septic shock or Sx)
- **Upper UTI is a common cause of sepsis or septic shock** (which can be informally called Urosepsis) & it should be highly considered in septic pts even w/o urinary Sx, especially for elderly w/ altered mental status. IV abx should be initiated w/ in 1 hr along w/ stat IV hydration (follow sepsis protocol)
- **Foley cath should be discontinued as soon as it is NOT indicated** due to an↑ risk of iatrogenic (preventable) UTI. Consider condom cath (still ↑ UTI risk x2 comparing to no cath at all but is still better than foley cath) or urinal to get accurate ins & outs as indicated.
- **UTI diagnosis can be challenging sometime:** for septic patients (w/ AMS & unknown dysuria hx) with mildly positive UA (like negative nitrate, weak + esterase, 5 WBC & +1 bacteria). In critical pts → empirically treat w/ abx while you pan-culture & look for another source of infx.

30. Volume Overload

A diagnosis of overloaded volume status can be elicited by a good h & p. It can be attributed to CHF (systolic mostly but also diastolic w/ preserved EF), cirrhosis, or nephropathy in most cases. In the in pt setting, volume overload is often iatrogenic caused simply by too much IV fluid or over-resuscitated truly hypovolemic pts (failure to adjust fluid infusion rate from replacement fluid deficit to maintenance rate). Often it is hard to assess volume status accurately.

History:
- **Ask about compliance w/ fluid restriction (1-1. 5 Liter) & ↓ Na⁺ diet,** especially for CHF pts. Any Na rich food & processed foods, salty foods may NOT necessarily taste salty to the pt. This is especially common during or around the holidays (eating at restaurants, canned foods, fried foods, etc).
- **Ask about meds compliance:** Have they skipped any doses of meds recently? Ask this question particularly to pts on diuretics who have complained about ↑ urinary frequency as a side effect. Also ask if they have been adjusting their Lasix or diuretic dose depending on their daily weight (Do they have scale at home)?
- **Have they taken or been prescribed any new meds recently?** One common culprit is NSAIDs (associated w/ worsening heart failure/HTN & of course worsening CKD).
- **Ask about missing dialysis** it is a common cause for volume overload & SOB/pulm edema hospital admissions. Always ask about recent weight change.

Exam & tests:
- Pts w/ volume status issues should be examined multiple times per day to assess the rate of

diuresis or IV fluid infusion in case of hypo or hypervolemia (stop when pt is euvolemic).

- **Vitals:** especially BP (HoTN indicates poor LV function while elevated BP maybe the reason for diastolic or systolic CHF exacerbation).
- **Inspection**: ↑ daily weight, pitting edema which must be assessed over a bony surface such as the shins or metatarsals, pronounced neck veins & elevated JVP (↑ Sen. & Spec.) & be on the alert for IV fluids hanging in the pt's room that are flowing continuously when in fact these fluids should have been held. Dependent edema is commonly seen in bedridden or supine pts in flank regions.
- **Auscultation**: Crackles & rales, shifting dullness from ascites, high liver span assessed via percussion, S3 heart sound due to turbulent blood flow from high volume (gallop)
- **CXR**: to establish a baseline w/ serial x-rays to assess improvement in the case of pulm edema (CXR changes occur quickly in comparison to PNA infiltrations). Remember to look at the CXR yourself to assess for Kerley B lines, hilar haze, cephalization of pulm vasculature, thickening of pleural fissures, peribronchial cuffing, diffuse opacification (AKA complete white out), & pleural effusion.
- **TTE**: should be considered up front to evaluate & compare ejection fraction or at least establish a baseline.
- **RUQ ultrasound**: to evaluate for hepatomegaly & congestion.
- **Labs:** Serum Cr (elevated Cr usually indicates renal involvement which could be either AKI or ESRD w/ missed HD) & BNP (elevated BNP indicates volume overload).

Management:
For all pts: stop IV fluids & consider mnemonic LMNOP (Lasix, Morphine, nitrates, O_2, posture), which is basically Tx for pulm edema (pt is sick & needs emergent Tx). Also, recommend a ↓ Na diet, fluid restriction, record daily ins & outs, encourage strict meds & HD compliance (if applicable).
For ESRD pts who have missed HD, arrange for dialysis, consult nephrology, & educate regarding compliance.
For cirrhosis pts w/ ascites, assess the need for therapeutic paracentesis & replace albumin (25 ml of albumin for every 2 liters of ascitic fluid removed).

Special considerations:

- **Pulmonary edema or congestion can occur w/o signs of peripheral edema** (lower extremities swelling, JVD, & hepatojugular reflex), especially if the etiology is HTN urgency/emergency w/ CHF & vice versa, peripheral edema can occur w/o pulm edema. The cornerstone of Tx is diuresis, especially for peripheral edema as these pts may sometimes have 10-20 liters of extra volume that needs to be eliminated.

> **Attention:** Pts w/ pulm edema from uncontrolled HTN w/o peripheral edema can be euvolumic (or even volume depleted from chronic diuresis) & diuresis should be brief along w/ controlling BP.

- **The physical examination** of pts who are volume depleted is often less telling than that of their overloaded counterparts.
- **Diuresis should be targeted** to achieve daily negative fluid balance. Net negative of 0.5-1L is usually safe, & might need to be more when

patient is symptomatic. Always check BMP (for K & Cr), Mg, & phosphate, & correct electrolyte abnormality as needed (Q 12 hrs). It is highly recommended to supplement K^+ & Mg^{2+} orally in the case of a high diuresis target, even if they are normal (prophylactically).

- **Usually loop diuresis w/ Lasix or Bumex either orally or IV** (PO meds do NOT absorb effectively due to intestinal edema in volume overload pts) is adequate. If the response is suboptimal, you can add thiazide diuretics like metolazone (once a day 30 minutes before the loop diuretic dose) for a synergetic effect.

- **Monitor serum Cr closely** as risk of AKI is a common consequence of overdiuresis. ↓diuretic dose (or even stop it) in case of Cr elevation (↓ urine output is another indicator for volume depletion). ↓central venous pressure (CVP) in ICU pts w/ a central line (normal CVP is 8-12) is a good sign of volume depletion (low CVP is almost always a sign of low volume status & indicating need for IV fluid).

> **Attention:** measure CVP "by yourself" as it is an essential value and you need it to be accurate.

- **NOT all edema or ascites needs diuresis** such as in the case of cirrhosis or malnutrition. In these cases, low oncotic pressure intravascularly causes "leakage" of the fluid into the interstitial space (third space). Pt's intravascular volume might be low & diuretics may NOT help. Measure CVP (if central line is available in the ICU) & urine Na. You may need to give IV fluid in the case of persistent low BP, ↓ CVP, ↓ urine Na^{+} & signs of poor end organ perfusion, such as AKI. Improving nutrition may ↓ the edema (albumin infusion is expensive & does NOT help due to the short half life).

31. Volume Depletion

Most cases of volume depletion can be attributed to an etiology of gastrointestinal losses, renal losses, skin losses, third space sequestration, or iatrogenic causes.

H & P:

- GI loss like diarrhea or vomiting? GI bleeding indicated by either BRBPR or black, tarry stool? ↓ PO fluid intake for any reason such as an elderly pt w/ AMS, NPO w/o IV fluid, or excessive sweating? Finally: consider pancreatitis, trauma such as crush injuries (Which could reveal pancreatic injury), recent surgery, or abdominal pain that could indicate peritonitis. All of these etiologies could contribute to third spacing.

- **Vitals→** tachycardia (first sign usually but maybe masked by AV node blocking agents) & HoTN. Tachypnea for any reason can ↑ insatiable water loss & cause volume depletion.

- Helpful equations to know:
  MAP=CO x TPR
  CO= HR x SV
  MAP= HR x SV x TPR
  HR= MAP/SV x TPR.

  (Mean artery pressure MAP, Cardiac output CO, Total peripheral resistance TPR, Heart rate HR, Stroke volume SV).

- **Inspection:** malaise, fatigue, thirst, muscle cramping, syncope, postural dizziness, abdominal & CP due to ischemia of the mesenteric or coronary vasculature, confusion, & altered mental status due to ↓ cerebral vascular perfusion. Assess skin turgor or lack thereof & delayed capillary refill. Tachypnea may be present due to acidosis. Muscular irritability (or cramps) & confusion may be present due to metabolic alkalosis. Muscle weakness & cramping may be observed due to hyperkalemia or hypokalemia. Seizures & coma may occur due to hyponatremia or hypernatremia. Flattened neck veins may be noted.

- **Auscultation**→Listen for groaning & moaning due to abdominal pain or CP as well as muscle cramping. Pts may tell you that they have been urinating more or even less frequently (due to AKI/ dehydration). Tachycardia & tachypnea may be present as mentioned above.

- **Labs: Check BMP** (elevated Cr usually indicates overdiuresis & intravascular volume depletion). Check **urine electrolytes** (urine Na & urine Cr along w/ BMP) & calculate **FeNa** (calculator **available online**) or **FeUrea** if pt is on diuresis (get urine Cr & urine Urea along w/ BMP). Calculate the **BUN to Cr ratio** (high in dehydration). Check **lactic acid** level to assess for lactic acidosis (usually q4-6hrs until resolution).

Management: IV hydration (mostly normal saline): start w/ few liters boluses (as needed) & then keep maintenance fluid (if can NOT tolerate PO).

Attention:
1. Dehydration is different than hypovolemia although they are treated mostly the same. Hypovolemia "low blood volume", which is NOT identical to dehydration "loss of water" because blood is NOT pure water.
2. FeNa (&even FeUrea) are very helpful to diagnose the etiology of **oliguria**. FeNa <1% → prerenal (Tx mostly w/ hydration) vs >1→renal/post-renal. FeNa is NOT very helpful in case of normal UOP.

32. Electrolyte imbalances

Hypernatremia

This always implies a free water deficit. It leads to neurological abnormalities, such as confusion, disorientation, seizure or even coma. Severity of Sx may vary depending on the chronicity of the hyponatremia.

Causes:
1. **Hypovolemia with Dehydration,** which is water loss more than Na (poor PO intake, diarrhea, DKA, elderly w/ AMS, fever, PNA or other types of insensible losses). Hypovolemia is different than dehydration due to the equal loss of water & Na in the former.
Tx is w/ volume expansion & fluid replacement. Rate of correction depends on the duration of hypernatremia.
2. **Normo- or hypervolemia hypernatremia**, such as **Diabetes Insipidus (DI):** There are two types: central & nephrogenic. Both give the following: ↓ urine osmolality, & ↑ urine volume.
a) Central DI is caused by a failure to produce antidiuretic hormone (ADH) in the brain. The pt will have a prompt ↑ in urine osmolarity w/ administration of DDAVP. Tx is w/ DDAVP (vasopressin).
b) Nephrogenic DI is caused by insensitivity of the kidney to ADH. Pt will have no change in both urine volume & osmolarity w/ DDAVP.

Tx is to correct the underlying cause (e.g. hypokalemia, hypercalcemia). Use thiazide diuretics for other causes.

Hyponatremia:

Hypo-osmolar (True) Hyponatremia
May present (similar to hypernatremia) w/ neurologic abnormalities, such as confusion, disorientation, seizures, or coma. The first step in management is to

assess volume status to determine the cause, & therefore, the Tx.

1. **Hypervolemic hyponatremia:** Pts w/ edema & swelling. Causes: Congestive heart failure (CHF), Nephrotic syndrome or Cirrhosis. Tx is to correct the underlying cause (& usually fluid restriction to <800cc/day). For CHF pts, hyponatremia is a prognostic marker for disease progression & usually does NOT need to be treated if it is asymptomatic & NOT severe (>120meq/L).

Tx: loop diuretics & optimize CHF meds to improve heart function (in CHF). Consider Albumin infusion (in cirrhosis).

2. **Hypovolemic hyponatremia: Causes:** Volume depletion (due to diuretics, vomiting, & diarrhea) **causes an appropriate ADH response** → ↑ water retention & Na level ↓. **Tx** is by correcting the underlying cause & normal saline replacement (to correct the volume & remove ADH stimulation). Remember to check serum Na frequently during replacement.

3. **Euvolemic hyponatremia:**
Causes:
- **SIADH (Syndrome of Inappropriate ADH)**: usually due to CNS problem or malignancy like small cell carcinoma in the lung. No volume deficits in SIADH. Tests: ↑ urine Na (>20 mEq/L), ↑ urine osmolality (>100 mOsm/Kg), ↓ serum osmolality (<290 mOsm/Kg), Normal Cr, BUN & Bicarbonate
- **Addison's disease** (insufficient aldosterone production): The key to this diagnosis is the presence of hyponatremia w/ **hyperkalemia & mild metabolic acidosis along w/ HoTN.** Treat w/ aldosterone replacement (fludrocortisone).

- **Hypothyroidism, psychogenic polydipsia, & hyperglycemia** (artificial "pseudo" drop in Na)

Tx:
- If mild or no Sx, treat by restricting fluids & managing the underlying problem.
- If moderate to severe or neurologic Sx, treat w/ the following: NS infusion w/ loop diuretics or Hypertonic 3% saline (which ↑ Na by 10meq/L for every one liter)
- Check serum Na frequently. Do NOT correct serum Na more than 10-12 mEq/L in the first 24 hrs. Correction rate can go up to 4-6meq/L in the first 6 hrs if severe Sx like seizure is present. Quick correction can cause permanent pontine osmotic demyelination & paralysis
- ADH blockers (conivaptan & tolvaptan) for refractory cases.

Hyperkalemia:
Common causes:
- Renal failure (prevents K excretion) w/ ↑ K diet or missing dialysis (for ESRD pts)
- Metabolic acidosis (↓ renal K excretion & transcellular shift out of the cells) & insulin deficiency, such as DKA
- Medicine: like K-sparing diuretics (such as spironolactone), digoxin toxicity, ACE inhibitors & ARBs (inhibit aldosterone), & β blockers (while β-agonists help in decreasing K; albuterol inhaler can be used for hyperkalemia)
- ↑ release from tissues such as muscles (e.g. rhabdomyolysis) or red blood cells (e.g. hemolysis).
- Adrenal aldosterone deficiency (Addison's disease), so check BP for HoTN
- Type IV renal Tubular Acidosis RTA (↓ aldosterone effect)
- Pseudohyperkalemia can occur for various reasons most commonly is delay in processing

the blood sample (hemolysis). Repeat blood test if you suspect hemolysis.

Management: First, you have to order EKG & look for peaked T-waves & cardiac arrhythmias.
Severe hyperkalemia or hyperkalemia w/ EKG abnormalities: such as peaked T waves, administer Ca gluconate IV (to protect the heart), & then administer regular insulin (10 u IV)& glucose (50% dextrose IV, 50ml) or Albuterol (nebulizer) to shift K into the cells. Along w/ addressing the underlying problem like stopping the offending meds, treat DKA, get dialysis, etc.
Mild-Moderate hyperkalemia (no EKG abnormalities), administer regular insulin, glucose (dextrose IV), & PO Kayexalate (to remove K from the body). Loop diuretics if pt makes urine. Correct causes for acidosis, rhabdomyolysis, & hemolysis. Bicarb is NOT very effective (do NOT use).

Hypokalemia:
Causes:
- Dietary insufficiency
- Diuretics (urinary loss)
- ↑ aldosterone (Conn's syndrome), causes HTN as well
- Vomiting (leads to metabolic alkalosis, which shifts K intracellularly, & volume depletion which ↑ aldosterone)
- Proximal (Type II) & distal (Type I) RTA
- Bartter syndrome (the defect here is similar to loop diuretics' mechanism) & Gitelman syndrome (similar to thiazide diuretics' mechanism)

Management: K replacement either PO or IV. Maybe both are needed especially in case of EKG changes (T wave flattening or any new arrhythmias) or severe hypokalemia. There is no maximum rate on PO K replacement, but IV K replacement must be slow so as to prevent an arrhythmia from overly rapid administration (peripheral 10mEq/hr, central 20mEq/hr). IV K also could be very vein irritating (burning sensation especially if small veins).

> **Attention:** Hypokalemia leads to cardiac rhythm disturbances (EKG can show "U-waves"), & it can also cause muscular weakness. This effect can be so severe that can cause rhabdomyolysis.

Hypomagnesaemia:
This presents w/ hypocalcaemia (Mg is required for PTH release), hypokalemia & cardiac arrhythmias.

Causes: Loop diuretics, alcohol abuse & drugs.

Tx: PO (GI irritation) or IV replacement depends on the severity.

Hypercalcemia:
Causes: The most common cause is primary hyperparathyroidism. Other causes include malignancy (PTHrP), granulomatous diseases (activate vitamin D), vitamin A & D intoxication, thiazide diuretics, tuberculosis, histoplasmosis, & berylliosis. Order malignancy work up for unexplained hypercalcemia.

Primary hyperparathyroidism: Most pts present w/ asymptomatic hypercalcemia. They may present w/ kidney stones, osteoporosis, osteomalacia, fractures, confusion, depression, constipation & abdominal pain. Labs show ↑ PTH & Ca. Tx is surgical removal in the following circumstances: any Symptomatic disease, renal insufficiency, markedly elevated 24-hr urine Ca or very elevated serum Ca (>12. 5)

Acute, severe hypercalcemia: The pt may present w/ confusion, constipation, nephrogenic DI (polyuria &

polydipsia), short QT syndrome on EKG, renal
insufficiency, ATN & kidney stones.

Management:
1. Hydration: ↑ volume of normal saline, about 3-4
liters **2. Calcitonin (Miacalcin):** 4IV/kg q12 hrs & repeat
PRN (usually acts fast)
3. Bisphosphonate IV (pamidronate) especially for
cancer related ↑ Ca (very potent but slow acting 2-
4days) **4.Steroids** if the etiology is granulomatous
disease. **Furosemide** is discouraged & should NOT be
used even though it can ↓ Ca.

Hypocalcaemia:
Causes: Surgical removal of the parathyroid gland,
hypomagnesaemia (Mg is required for PTH release)
Vitamin D deficiency, acute hyperphosphatemia
(phosphate binds Ca & lowers it), fat malabsorption (fat
binds Ca in the gut & prevents absorption), PTH
resistance: pseudohypoparathyroidism that
accompanies a short fourth finger, round face, & mental
retardation.

Presentation & management: Severe hypocalcemia
presents w/ seizures, neural twitching (Chvostek's sign &
Trousseau's sign), & arrhythmia (prolonged QT on
EKG). Replace Ca IV (Ca gluconate 1-2 gr IV) or PO
($CaCo_3$ = TUMS) depending on severity. Treat the
underlying problem (phosphate binder like Renagel for
hyperphosphatemia, pancreatic enzymes for fat
malabsorption in case of chronic pancreatitis, etc). Give
activated Vitamin D for ESRD pts (like Calcitriol)

Special considerations:
- **Hypomagnesemia** can cause renal loss of K &
  "refractory" hypokalemia. Replete both
  electrolytes Mg & K together (in addition to the
  Ca as it also interferes w/ their levels in case of
  deficiency).

- **During Tx of DKA** you should replenish K even though it is normal. DKA management protocol from American Diabetes Association states that if K level is between 3. 3-5.3 give 20-30 mEq in each liter of IV fluid to keep serum K between 4 & 5 mEq/L.
- **Each 10 mEq K you give, total serum K will ↑by 0. 1 mEq/L** (IV replace the same as oral).
- **In case of hypocalcemia, check albumin level.** Total Ca concentration will change in parallel to the albumin concentration (because part of the Ca is bound to albumin). In general, the serum Ca concentration falls by 0. 8 mg/dL (0. 2 mmol/L) for every 1. 0 g/dL (10 g/L) fall in the serum albumin concentration (less than 4. 0 g/L). Ionized Ca does NOT need albumin correction (more expensive test usually ordered in critical pts & Symptomatic hypocalcemia)
- **Online calculator for free water deficits for hypernatremia** (depends on body weight, Na level, gender, etc) can calculate how much total free water you need to give. Usually D5 w/ ½ or ¼ NS is preferred for IV correction or free water flushes through NG or PEG tube.
- **Caution w/ quick correction of hypernatremia** (cerebral edema), especially if NOT Symptomatic (safe correction rate is 10 meq/L in 24hrs). Check Na level in 4-6 hrs from the time fluids are started & adjust the fluid rate as needed (check other electrolytes as well & correct as needed)
- **Hyperphosphatemia is common in CKD/ESRD pts.** Tx w/ either Ca-based binder like Ca acetate or non-Ca binder like Renagel (if hypercalcemia is an issue). Ca x PhO4 product >55 ↑ the probability for metastatic calcification in pts w/ ESRD & contribute to substantial amount of morbidity & mortality (recognize & treat early w/ phosphate binder).

Neurology

33. Falls, syncope, & loss of consciousness

While working as a resident you will probably get some calls about a pt that fell out of bed or fell while getting up. The first thing to do is to find out why the pt fell.

Evaluation for pt who recently fell:
- Determine if there is any head trauma, if so consider CT head to check for IC bleeding (you can defer that in case of absence of concerning signs like N/V, HAs, LOC, focal neuro deficits, anticoagx), look for scalp lacerations.
- Examine pt for extremity trauma (pain w/ passive range of motion), get x-ray (prn). Pay special attention to hip fractures in elderly pts.
- Make sure adequate fall precautions are in place (to protect pt from pulling lines/foley & hurt him/herself or others) & consider 1:1 sitter (or even restraints as the last resort) if applicable.
-

Syncope & Loss of Consciousness (LOC): Syncope is a transient, self-limited LOC due to acute global impairment of cerebral blood f low w/ rapid onset, brief duration & generally, complete spontaneous recovery.

Causes of syncope (& LOC) are divided into three categories	
1. Neurally mediated	Vasovagal syncope
2. Cardiac	Structural problems like aortic stenosis or arrhythmias
3. Orthostatic hypotension	Due to volume depletion or meds

Common causes of Syncope & LOC:
- **Vasovagal:** "situational syncope", is very common & can occur during embarrassing

situations, blood draws, coughing, urination (micturition syncope), or defecation (good prognosis in general)

- **Arrhythmia:** can be due to tachy-arrhythmias, bradycardia, arrhythmias or heart blocks (diagnose w/ EKG, holter for 24-48 hrs, or event monitor for 30 days depending on the frequency of the Sx)
- **Structural heart disease:** includes LOC from ischemic heart disease such as a MI, hypertrophic cardiomyopathy, acute aortic dissection, pericardial tamponade, & aortic stenosis (consider TTE, ECG, CXR & CTA as indicated)
- **Orthostatic HoTN:** associated w/ movement from lying or sitting position to standing. More common in elderly. Causes: volume depletion (like GI bleed & dehydration), autonomic dysfunction as in DM pts.
- **Neurologic:** can be due to CVA (NOT commonly causing syncope as the infarction needs to be really large in order to affect the alertness), hyperventilation, & seizures (consider head CT or EEG).

> **Attention:** CVA "in general" does NOT cause syncope, unless it envolves the brainstem or both himospheres (which are rare).

- **Meds:** various meds such as β blockers (causing bradycardia), diuretics, vasodilators (orthostatic hypotensive syncope) can cause syncope
- **Hypoglycemia** (from excessive insulin or postprandial after heavy meal in pre-diabetic condition), **carotid stenosis, & acute blood loss.**

History: Why did the pt fall? Tripped or felt dizzy? Where pt landed? Any eyewitnesses? Was there complete loss of consciousness? Any previous episodes of syncope? Duration of loss of consciousness? Did the pt recover spontaneously, completely & w/o consequences (like in cardiac cause) or was confused for a while (postictal state like post-seizure)? Did the pt lose postural tone? Bowel or bladder control? Associated Sx & hx before or after syncopal episode? Any "aura" before event or N/V, warmth, pallor, lightheadedness, & /or diaphoresis? Any pre-existing conditions, meds, family hx?

Work up for Syncope/LOC:
- Obtain full hx, vitals including orthostatic BP (if systolic BP dropped >20 or diastolic >10 from supine to standing position after 3 minutes from standing)
- Tilt table test (may be positive w/ orthostatic/postural syncope secondary to autonomic dysfunction)
- Review meds (β blockers, Ca channel blockers, diuretics, pain/psychiatric meds)
- Check labs (CBC/CMP), EKG, TTE (if cardiac source is suspected)
- Holter or event monitor if arrhythmia in differential, carotid US, especially in elderly, head CT/MRI if neurogenic in differential

Special consideration:
- 1st non-cardiac syncope has a good prognosis & unlikely that it will reoccur.
- Assess the need of resuming anticoagx & discuss w/ the pt & the family (weight risk & benefits) in case of a fib, DVT, pulm embolism, etc w/ recurrent falls (or bleeding). Sometimes risks highly outweigh benefits & stopping anticoagx should be considered.

- Recommend safe environment for pts after their 1st syncope or seizure episode for at least 6months & observe for recurrence. Caution with operating heavy machinery, ladder climbing, driving, swimming, etc.

Syncope vs. Seizure

Feature	Syncope	Seizure
Aura	N/V & diaphoresis (vagal or parasympathetic Sx)	Unusual behavior including automatism (like lips smacking)
Convulsions	Usually short (<10second)	Variable
Postictal state	No	Yes
Others	Skin pallor & clamminess	Tongue bites & incontinence

Compare syncope & seizure, as they can be similar

34. Altered Mental Status (AMS)

Acute change in level of consciousness & /or cognition.

Delirium: Clouded consciousness, waxing & waning, agitation, hallucinations, paranoia, ↑ sympathetic activity & usually reversible causes (mostly in an in pt setting). It can be hypo or hyperactive delirium.
Dementia: Chronic process of reduced cognition, primarily w/ memory. Though unlike delirium, attention & alertness are preserved until late stages.

Differential diagnosis:
↑ insurance billing to level 5 due to the broad DDx.

Metabolic Abnormalities:
- Electrolyte abnormalities: hypo/hypernatremia, hypo/hyperglycemia, hypercalcemia, acidosis/alkalosis; (K+ abnormalities do NOT cause delirium)
- Encephalopathy: hyperammonemia in liver disease, uncontrolled HTN, renal failure/uremia, hypoxia/hypercapnia
- Endocrine abnormalities: thyroid storm, myxedema coma, adrenal crisis
- Nutritional derangements: Vitamin B12 deficiency, thiamine deficiency (Wernicke's or Beriberi)

Neurologic Abnormalities
- Structural: tumor/mass effect, herniation, hemorrhage, infarct, abscess, normal pressure hydrocephalus (wet, wacky & wobbly)
- Seizure disorders (postictal state)
- B12 deficiency (Subacute combined degeneration)

Infection
- Sepsis, PNA, UTI (especially in elderly)
- Meningitis/encephalitis
- HIV encephalopathy (mainly is subacute) & Neurosyphilis (test blood for RPR).

Meds/Toxins
- Sedatives, hypnotics, narcotics, street drugs
- Benzodiazepines in the elderly
- Narcotic pain meds (recent changes/additions); adverse reaction to narcotic meds is pt-specific (based on age, renal, & liver function)
- Anti-cholinergics (always consider Benadryl in elderly)
- Alcohol (DTs)/benzodiazepine/barbiturate withdrawal
- Steroids
- Anti-convulsants (e.g. Dilantin)
- Anti-depressant
- Anti-hypertensive (HoTN causing ↓ cerebral blood flow)
- Anti-psychotics (e.g. Haldol & Seroquel)

Systemic abnormalities
- Decompensated CHF
- Acute urinary retention, especially in elderly
- Anemia
- Hypo/hyperthermia, hypoperfusion, hypoventilation
- Constipation (common reason for AMS in elderly)

Psychiatric Abnormalities: like mania/depression
Trauma: brain concussion

H & P:
History: Obtain event hx from the pt, nursing staff & /or family

- Timing, trauma, setting, precipitating factors, aura/prodrome (role/out epilepsy)
- Past medical hx, social hx (EtOH abuse→give Ativan as per CIWA protocol)
- New or change in meds (stop morphines, benzos, anticholinergics, etc)

Physical Exam:
- Vitals: Hypo/hyperthermia, hypo/HTN, respiratory rate, tachycardia/bradycardia & SaO_2
- Level of alertness
- Pupil size & reflex (e.g., cocaine or opioids)
- Cranial nerves (looking for signs of stroke), carotid bruit (a possible source of a stroke), nuchal rigidity (meningitis)
- Arrhythmia/murmur (stroke, ↓ blood flow, new onset murmur/arrhythmia indicating underlying heart pathology)
- Air movement, crackles (hypoxia, PNA, etc.)
- Ascites, asterixis, abdominal tenderness (constiptation could cause AMS in elderly), petechiae, jaundice (liver failure)
- Suprapubic tenderness/bladder distension (UTI, urinary retention)
- Signs suggestive of basilar skull fracture: Battle's sign (discoloration over mastoid process), Raccoon eyes (discoloration around the eyes)
- Spontaneous movements, response to noxious stimuli, & posture.

Stabilize Pt based on findings from hx/physical/ACLS protocol, if trauma to spinal cord suspected, do NOT move the pt (risk of permanent paralysis).
Work-up based on differential obtained from pt specific hx/physical findings:
- CBG, ABG/CXR, EKG/cardiac enzymes, CBC/CMP, TSH, B12, FOLATE, RPR, Ammonia level

- Head CT- w/o contrast, lumbar puncture, EEG
- UDS, anticonvulsant level, digoxin level, EtOH level
- UA, urine culture, blood culture/gram stain, bladder scan, CXR

Special consideration:
- **"Quick assessment"** for AMS: check the following "automatically" when you are evaluating AMS & correct the abnormal: Vitals, CBC, CMP, ABG (prn), CXR (prn), meds review (Always; hold sedating/psych meds), review admitting diagnoses & PMH. R/o sepsis/ infx, polypharmacy, exacerbating existed diagnoses (phsych or organic illness).
- **Tx directed towards the underlying disorder** (do NOT just give Haldol or benzos w/o initial evaluation). Try non-pharmacological methods like opening blinds in the morning, get the pts their glasses/hearing aids, turn the TV on in the AM & off in the PM, limit blood withdrawal in the PM, etc.
- **Olanzapine is better for agitation in elderly** (& it can be used to prevent delirium in elderly before surgeries like for hip replacement). Benzodiazepines can cause paroxysmal agitation instead of sedation.
- **Wrists restraints** are indicated if pt is agitated & is at risk of harming himself/herself or others.
- **Always follow ACLS algorithm for unstable pts** & do a quick exposure head to toe looking for signs of trauma, drug patches (like fentanyl), infectious sources (lines/devices/caths).
- **Being in the ICU is a cause of "ICU delirium/agitation"** (r/o other organic delirium causes before calling it ICU delirium). There is some evidence that delirium can be prevented. Outside the ICU, repeated reorientation, noise reduction, cognitive stimulation, vision & hearing

aids, adequate hydration, & early mobilization can reduce the incidence of delirium in hospitalized patients. Olanzapine (or even Haloperidol) prophylaxis in patients undergoing hip surgery reduced the severity & duration of delirium. Among patients in the ICU, the duration of delirium was significantly ↓ w/ early mobilization & interruptions in sedation.

- **CVA**: can manifest in many ways including AMS. Order CT scan head w/o contrast to r/o intracranial bleeding or early signs of ischemia (like tissue edema which probably means that CVA happened >6hrs) & consider IV tPA if time between symptoms & IV tPA is <3-4.5 hrs (consult neurology). Ischemic CVA Tx is usually just secondary risk factor prevention like control HTN (keep it elevated but <160/90 in the first 1-2 days), DM, HLD. Work up is usually the same & mostly in pt (MRI, transcranial & carotid Doppler, TTE, lipid panel, etc).

Attention: Transient Ischemic Attack TIA is a "minor stroke" last for minutes to hours (<24h, mostly one hour) from the Sx. Work up is similar to CVA (ASAP) due to high risk of recurrence in the next 1-2 days.

Seizure: tonic-clonic, partial, absence, etc. Chronic management is usually by neurology but acute Tx is essential by medicine service. **Acute Tx: Benzos** (like Ativan 2-4mg IV q2-3 min or Versed drip) is a 1st line Tx, you can give bolus or drip if the seizure is refractory. **Fosphenytoin** IV (18mg/kg bolus) is a 2nd line (also consider **phenobarbital** IV w/ intubation w/ or w/o sedation w/ **propofol** as a last resort). Loading dose of **Keppra or dilantin** can follow the Benzos (for pts w/ hx of seizures) until neurology give further help. NO long-term Tx is recommended for 1st time unprovoked seizure (low % of recurrence, unless there is CNS lesions like CVA, bleeding, mass or trauma) or abnormal MRI or EEG (treat after 1st seizure). **Common seizure etiology:** old CVA (usually >6 months), brain tumor (primary or secondary), & trauma. **Tests:** CT scan, MRI, & EEG (last two are standard of care for all seizure pts). **Provoked seizures:** needs to Tx the etiology w/o anti-epilepsy meds. Common etiologies: electrolytes abnormalities (↑↓ Na, ↑↓ glucose, ↑↓ Ca), drugs (like Ecstasy), CNS lesions, EtOH withdrawal, or CNS infx. Monitor any 1st seizure for 6 months & advise to avoid driving, climbing ladders, swimming, operating heavy machinery, etc.

Attention: if pt had few interrupted seizures episodes at the same day→ still one seizure.
Attention: if pt did not wake up in between seizures→ possible subclinical non-convulsion seizures (do EEG)→ urgent Tx (benzos).

35. Headaches (HA)

HA is pain or discomfort in the head, scalp, or neck which can be benign to life threatening, depending on the cause of the HA. Always obtain a good hx & physical exam when it comes to HAs. Always evaluate the pt at the bedside, especially if it is a new complaint. ***Alarming findings (proceed w/ imaging instead of symptomatic management):*** *1st or the worst HA, progressive in hours to days, recurrent, changed from previous, systemic Sx like weight loss or fever (indicate inflammatory or malignant cause) or abnormal physical exam.*

Differential diagnosis & Management:

Medicine: cause HAs like Vasodilators (NTG, β blockers, nifedipine, ACE inhibitors, hydralazine), chemotherapeutic drugs, transplant meds, abx (tetracyclines, amphotericin, griseofulvin, sulfonamides, chloroquine), & others (EtOH, cocaine, carbon monoxide, caffeine withdrawal, estrogen withdrawal, progestin, tamoxifen, & SSRIs). Paradoxically, pain relieving meds overuse/misuse can cause HAs & Tx → stop the offending agent.

Migraine: More common in females & peaks between the 20-50 years. Two types of migraines: **classic migraine** (unilateral/throbbing HA, N/V, photo/phonophopia, *w/* aura) & **common migraine** (all previous but **w/o** aura). The most common trigger is stress (ask about any other trigger & advise to avoid it & instruct to keep headache diary). **First-line abortive meds for migraines include**: ASA, acetaminophen, NSAIDs (e.g. ibuprofen, Diclofenac), & consider any triptan meds (if refractory & check cardiac & neuro contraindication) like sumatriptan (5HT1D agonist) either PO, IV, or nasal (one dose q 1 hour x 2), will usually work in aborting 90% of migraines. Tramadol (as well as narcotics) is also effective in aborting migraine (use as last resort especially if sumatriptan is contraindicated). If N/V → Phenergan (especially good for migraine pts). Avoid triptans in pts w/ CAD disease, variant angina, uncontrolled HTN, & during pregnancy. **Prophylaxis:** Consider prophylactic therapy for frequent attacks that have significant impact on pt's lifestyle (>2 episodes a month). Medicine used: β blockers (propranolol), CCBs (nifedipine & verapamil), Topamax (it is anticonvulsant & can help in weight loss), Pizotifen (5HT antagonist), TCAs (amitriptyline) & others.

Meningitis:
- Fever & neck stiffness usually present (± AMS)
- Generalized HA, which radiates to the neck
- Constant & severe; occasionally may begin abruptly
- Aggravated by flexion of the neck - **Brudzinski's sign** (flexing the neck causes flexion of the hips & knees); **Kernig's sign** (pain w/ flexing the hip at 90° & then trying to fully extend the knee; high false positive rate)
- Diagnosed w/ urgent LP & treated w/ urgent IV abx if **bacterial** (**CSF:** low Glucose -0.4 of blood glucose-, high protein & WBC ->500-w/ neutrophil predominance). **Tx:** Vanc + Rocephin IV); Symptomatic Tx if **viral** (WBC -<300- w/ lymph predominance, mild protein elevation & normal glocuse). Conisder **Steroids** in bacterial meningitis & get ID help if available.

> **Attention:** "Partially treated meningitis" is when the pt gets abx before the LP and CSF may not show a common CSF bacterial infx findings (elevated WBC & protein and low glucose). Consider abx until CSF culture is negative.

Tension HA (Non-vascular)
- Typically symmetrical bilateral tightness, non-pulsating quality,
- Tends to last for hrs & recurs each day, mild to moderate intensity
- Often associated w/ cervical dysfunction & stress or tension; no N/V or photophobia, 75% of pts are females

Management:
- Counseling & relevant advice
- Massage of the affected area w/ soothing analgesic rub
- Advise stress reduction, relaxation therapy & yoga or meditation
- Meds - ASA or acetaminophen, discourage stronger analgesics
- Avoid tranquilizers & antidepressants if possible.

Cluster HA: Occurs in paroxysmal clusters (hence the name) for weeks to months, & then completely remit for months to years (male>female). They typically occur at night, usually in the early hrs of the morning, though can occur at other times. Pts experience an intense pain around one eye or side of the head, & often the sclera becomes injected. They can have tearing & rhinorrhea on that side. They can also have swelling of the eye & drooping of the eyelid. There are no visual disturbances or vomiting.

Management:

Acute attack (brief Tx seldom effective): 100% O2 @10 L/min, sumatriptan, metoclopramide + dihydroergotamine IV or IM.

Prophylaxis (once a cluster starts): consider dihydroergotamine (take at night during a cluster); methysergide, prednisolone taper, lithium, verapamil, indomethacin (helps confirm diagnosis if there is response).

Temporal Arteritis (TA, giant cell arteritis): There is usually a persistent unilateral throbbing HA in the temporal region & scalp sensitivity/tenderness w/ localized thickening. TA may also involve the intracranial vessels, especially the ophthalmic artery causing optic atrophy & unilateral blindness (usually irreversible). Other Sx that should give you a high suspicion for TA when seen w/ the temporal HA include malaise, fatigue, low-grade fever, anorexia & weight loss, myalgias or arthralgias, & jaw claudication (pain on chewing).

Diagnosis is usually clinical w/ ESR usually elevated (often >100 mm/hr), biopsy w/ artery wall inflammation/granuloma confirms the diagnosis (though it can be normal as the lesions are focal in nature). Get biopsy (multiple required) if the clinical picture is NOT clear. MRI has ↑ sensitivity & specificity.

Tx: TA is very responsive to high-dose corticosteroids (prednisolone 60 mg/day w/ tapered doses). Start Tx immediately w/ ↑ suspicion to prevent permanent blindness (do NOT wait for ESR & biopsy results). Monitor clinical status, ESR, & CRP.

Hypertensive HA: Occurs in severe HTN such as malignant HTN or hypertensive encephalopathy. It is typically occipital. Throbbing HA is more severe upon waking in the morning. Treat the HTN & the HA will resolve.

Frontal Sinusitis: The HA of frontal sinusitis can be a diagnostic problem especially in the absence of, or lapse in time since, an obvious upper respiratory infx or vasomotor rhinitis. Some pts do NOT have hx of a preceding respiratory infx nor have signs of nasal obstruction or fever. Sinusitis is a relatively uncommon source of HA. It presents typically as a frontal or retro-orbital HA.

Diagnosis: tenderness over the frontal sinus & pain on percussion. Fever & edema of the upper eyelid may be present.

Tx: drain the sinus conservatively using steam inhalations. Abx: amoxicillin/clavulanate, cefaclor or doxycycline, & analgesics.

Post-lumbar puncture HA: Common; usually worsens w/ standing or sitting, & rapidly improves w/ lying flat; possibly due to CSF leakage. It can be severe w/ N/V, but resolution occurs w/ in 2-7 days.
Tx includes bed rest/hydration until resolution. If it persists (>5days), an epidural blood patch (by anesthesia) is recommended.

Benign Intracranial HTN (pseudotumor cerebri):
Typically occurs in young obese women & is usually associated w/ N/V. Papilledema will be present. However, CT & MRI scans are normal (hence *pseudo*tumor). However, LP reveals high CSF opening pressure, & normal CSF analysis. Often times the pt feels better after lumbar puncture because of CSF loss & ↓ in pressure. Linked to some drugs: tetracyclines (most common), nitrofurantoin, PO contraceptives, & Vitamin A.
Tx: Weight reduction & diuretics. Diamox (acetazolamide) is the 1st line Tx. However, acetazolamide has a Class C pregnancy risk. Corticosteroids are 2nd line. The Tx of choice to relieve Sx is repeated lumbar puncture.

SAH (Subarachnoid Hemorrhage):
SAH is a life-threatening event that should NOT be over looked at the primary care level due to high mortality rate. It manifests as sudden onset HA (moderate to intense severity- often described as the "worst HA of my life"). It is often referred to as the "thunderclap HA" because of its sudden onset. Localized at first (usually occipital) then generalized, pain & stiffness of the neck, vomiting & confusion/loss of consciousness. Neurological deficits may include hemiplegia (if intracerebral bleed) & third nerve palsy ("down & out" eye w/ a drooping of the eyelid).

> **Attention**: Occipital HA + vomiting + neck stiffness →SAH until proven otherwise.

Management:
- If the pt is having confusion/loss of consciousness, remember ABCs & assess the need for intubation. Consult neurosurgery immediately, & be wary of increasing ICP, as the risk for herniation is high if you attempt LP. You can use osmotic agents, such as mannitol & loop diuretics (Lasix) to ↓ ICP. Using IV steroids to control brain edema is controversial. If the pt is hypertensive, use IV β blockers.
- Neurological exam looking for any deficits
- Labs: order a CBC, CMP, Coagx panel, blood type & screen, cardiac enzymes, & an ABG
- Urgent head CT w/o contrast
- Lumbar puncture after CT (if you suspect a bleed, always do CT first in case of elevated ICP). It will show xanthochromia (yellowish tint) & elevated RBCs in the CSF analysis.
- Nimodipine is a good BP lowering agent for SAH pts

Cervical Spondylosis: HA from neck disorders caused by abnormalities in any structure innervated by the upper cervical nerves. Pain from cervical structures can be referred retro-orbitally & over one-half of the head. The pain usually starts from the occipital region w/ possible radiation to skull & facial area. It is usually present during movement & settles during resting. There is usually hx of trauma w/ associated features include stiffness & grating of the neck.
On examination there is usually tenderness to palpation over cervical vertebrae.
Management: Neck X-ray & MRI can help diagnosis. Physiotherapy modalities: hydrotherapy, muscle energy therapy, mobilization, manipulation (from experts) &

neck exercises (very important), supportive pillow, NSAIDs, neurosurgery consultation.

36. Pain

Is often considered the fifth vital sign. It is one of the most common complaints of pts admitted in the hospital & often, incorrectly managed. It is a subjective sensation & hence, hard to reliably quantify.

Classification & Management: Pain can be measured by VAS scale (0-10, 10 being the worst). Mild (1-3) usually needs Tylenol/NSAIDs, moderate (4-7) usually needs oral opioids (Percocet or lortab)/tramadol (w/ or w/o Tylenol/ NSAIDs) & severe (8-10) usually needs IV opioids. As pain is very subjective & pain tolerance is different; above formulas can be adjusted accordingly. Another classification is the chronicity of the pain (acute or chronic)

A. **Acute pain** (Postoperative pain, inflammation, trauma, burns, & sickle cell crisis): Usually lasts for a few days. Try to eliminate the source before starting the pt on a pain meds regimen. 1st line agents are non-narcotic analgesics such as acetaminophen & non-steroidal anti-inflammatory drugs (NSAIDs). They are most effective for mild to moderate pain, pain related to inflammation, musculoskeletal pain, & HAs. All NSAIDs inhibit cyclooxygenase (COX), usually both 1 & 2. The COX-1 enzyme is also expressed in the epithelium of the GI tract & hence, non-selective COX inhibitors can cause GI toxicity (ulcers & gastritis; take after food). There are non-selective COX-2 inhibitors, such as Celecoxib, but they are rarely used due to the ↑ risk of adverse cardiovascular events. Chronic use of COX-2 inhibitors has been reported to ↑ death from myocardial infarction. Some have IV formulations. Two of these IV formulations include IV ketorolac & IV acetaminophen, which are effective in avoiding or reducing the requirement of opioids.

Adverse effects: GI irritation, interstitial nephritis, NSAIDs nephropathy (including AKI due to inhibition of renal prostaglandins), & HTN w/ chronic use (Naproxen is maybe the safest). **Use w/ caution:** acetaminophen in hepatic impairment (use lower doses, usually <2 g/day). **Contraindications of NSAIDs usage:** renal insufficiency, CHF (still used/ Naproxin is preferred), GI bleed (or recent hx w/ caution), post-operative state (most of them, except Tylenol have an anti-platelet effect & also delay wound healing).

B. **Chronic pain (Cancer, terminal illness, neuropathic pain, & certain pain syndromes such as fibromyalgia):** Pts in continuous pain require round-the-clock analgesia. Usually long-acting opioids are give n at a basal dose w/ short-acting ones given as needed (PRN) at 10-20% of the basal dose. If frequent PRN doses are used, they should be added up & a new basal dose is calculated.

Opioids: Inadequate dosing w/ opioids is one of the most common errors made by physicians & leads to unnecessary suffering. Also, there is reluctance to use opioids due to unsubstantiated fear of addiction when evidence points out the fact that use of opioids for a genuine cause of pain rarely fosters addiction. Also, the physician should develop an opioid management plan or 'pain contract' w/ pts (mostly in out pt setting). This typically includes stipulations that pain meds will NOT be sought elsewhere, pt will abstain from illicit drugs, will keep clinic appointments as scheduled, & will obtain random urine drug screens.

A copy of this signed document is given to the pt & reviewed periodically during follow-up visits. Usually short-acting opioids such as morphine, Percocet (oxycodone/acetaminophen), loratab (hydrocodone/acetaminophen) are preferred in acute pain. Long-acting formulations such as MS Contin, Oxycontin controlled release, methadone, fentanyl patches (NOT preferred as 1st line) are reserved for chronic pain.

Adjuvant pain therapy:

- **Anticonvulsants** (gabapentin, pregabalin & valproate) & anti-depressants (amitriptyline, desipramine, duloxetine & venlafaxine) are considered 1st line drugs in neuropathic pain. Tricyclic anti-depressants are usually avoided because of adverse effects, mostly their anticholinergic effects. Gabapentin is usually started 1st (start w/ small dose & titrate up).
- **Muscle relaxant** like flexeril, Suboxone & baclofen (avoid driving car while on them) are preferred to treat muscle spasms in the neck, Back & extremities. Muscle pain usually is severe, non- radiating & associated usually w/ hrs to days hx of heavy lifting or excessive exercise. NSAIDs also can be used along w/ topical pain creams (like Diclofenac topical, Lidocaine patch, & Capsaicin cream) & hot massage.
- Consider **Physical therapy PT & exercise programs** (especially aquatic therapy for elderly w/ balance issues) for chronic pain like Fibromyalgia & chronic pain syndrome, as it can be very effective w/ Cognitive therapy. PT can also strengthen the muscles around the joints & ↓ osteoarthritis pain (especially knees & back pain)

Special consideration:

- **Addiction:** Opioid drug abuse is a common problem & steps must be taken by every health care professional to curb it. Pain meds should be prescribed by one health care practitioner & the pt must be bound by a "pain contract".

Judicious use of opioids & making every effort to wean pts off them would go a long way in dealing w/ this issue (narcotics prescribed for any reason ↑ mortality comparing to normal population).

> **Attention**: scheduled pain meds are preferred over "PRN" in order to ↓ addiction & ↑ efficacy. Add "PRN" at the top of scheduled meds in specific cases. Educate pt that pain may not go to zero &<3 is maybe acceptable in chronic pain.

- **Pt-controlled analgesia PCA:** a system through which the pt self-administers predetermined doses of opioids. Morphine & dilaudid are two commonly used drugs for PCA, & is usually used in pts requiring large doses of opioids, such as those w/ chronic pain syndromes, like sickle cell disease. PCA can administer a basal dose (at a continuous hourly rate) & bolus doses (which is administered by the pt) w/ a lockout interval (which can be adjusted, usually from 7-20 minutes). Advantages of a PCA include greater pain relief, pt satisfaction, & fewer complications.
- **Always prevent ileus/constipation** by starting bowel regimen (colace, Miralax, ± stimulants like Senna). Relistor (Methylnaltrexone) is an opioid reversal agent in the GI system (expensive; try to avoid the need for it). Urinary retention is an opioid side effect like constipation but maybe less common (NOT preventable).
- **Respiratory suppression** is an opioid side effect & it happen due to hypoventilation (↓ respiratory rate); so SOB & O_2 desaturation should be assessed in pts on opioids. Respiratory rate of 30-40 may NOT indicate an

opioid overdose. In general: avoid meds can ↓ mental status (like benzos or opioids) in pts who has respiratory distress or O_2 desaturation (for any reason) to avoid the need for intubation. Narcan is the opioid antidote (fast response).

- **Oxycodone** (w/o the Tylenol) has a high street value & drug abusers can use it by sniffing & IV for euphoria effects
- **Conversion of opioids** derivatives from type to another & from route to another (PO →IV or IV →PO) is **available online**. Chronic opioid users may need more than the calculated IV dose when converting from PO due to tolerance. Starting opioid doses should be lower for elderly.
- **Fentanyl** is NOT preferred for narcotic Naïve pts. **Methadon** has a lot of formulas (like tablets, oral solution, IV,etc) & it is common in hospice care.
- **Opioids rotation:** means changing the opioid type over time to ↓ side effect with prolonged use.

Geriatric

37. Geriatric medicine

Physiological (normal) Changes of Aging:

- Temperature: as one ages, fat stores & metabolic rates ↓, resulting in a tendency toward hypothermia
- Fluid Balance: total body water is reduced, thirst sensation blunted; therefore, elderly have higher risk for dehydration
- Hearing loss & changes in vision occur
- ↑ tendency for hypothyroidism & Vit D deficiency
- Atherosclerosis (up to 50% of people of both sexes have some degree of coronary artery disease CAD)
- ↑ tendency for gastroparesis
- ↓ in estrogen; ↑ in LH, FSH & vaginal atrophy
- ↓ in testosterone, ↓ libido, depression & Immune system slower to respond
- Muscle mass ↓ (consider chronic kidney disease CKD even if serum Cr is relatively low for pts w/ ↓ muscle mass or elderly & adjust meds doses to eGFR)
- Osteopenia/Osteoporosis & ↑ tendency toward fractures, especially hip or vertebral
- ↓ in pain perception, impaired reflexes & ↑ in reaction time (refer pt to DMV to reassess the ability to drive if you concern about being risk for themselves or others)
- ↓ quality of sleep due to ↑ night-time awakening, shorter REM stage & early morning wake up (but normal falling asleep)

Approach to Illness in Geriatric Population:
- Be mindful of **atypical presentations** of common illnesses in elderly. For example, an elderly pt w/ UTI may present w/ acute altered

mental status/confusion instead of fever & suprapubic discomfort

- Isolation, progressive loss of interest in conversation, loss of ability to complete ADLs independently, poor appetite & poor PO intake can all be signs of underlying dementia/delirium or depression
- **Common Problems in Elderly:**

Gait instability & Frequent falls: assess how often & situation (like dizziness which needs a full work up sometime or just mechanical like tripping on a carpet or a grandson), Head injury/LOC (especially if pt is on blood thinner, consider stopping them if risks overweight benefits), Previous fractures, review meds (possible dizziness from polypharmacy) & EtOH/drug abuse (get UDS). Consider Head CT if falls, urinary incontinence & recent changes in memory are present to r/o Normal Pressure Hydrocephalus NPH.

Orthostatic HoTN (consider ↓ BP meds doses even if the BP is normal if the pt has orthostatic Sx or dizziness as BP in elderly is acceptable around 130-140 systolic)

Neglect & Elder Abuse: needs high suspicion, consider nursing home placement & social worker help if the insurance allows.

Miscellaneous:
- Polypharmacy
- Failure to thrive
- Undiagnosed BPH & nocturia (↑ risk for falls)
- Depression (Screen w/ SIGECAPS & use SSRIs as it is "elderly friendly")
- Dementia: Impairment in short- & long-term memory & at least 1 of the

following: Impairment in abstract thinking, impaired judgment, Other disturbances of higher cortical function (agnosia, anomia, & visuospatial difficulties) & Personality change. Most common etiology for dementia is Alzhaimer or vascular (chronic ischemia). **"Normal" short-term memory loss is common in elderly** but it will NOT cause daily activity impairment (pt basically can still drive/shop/cook/manage finance but they have difficulty remembering grandchild's name, etc)

- Delirium/Acute Agitation & Incontinence are also common.

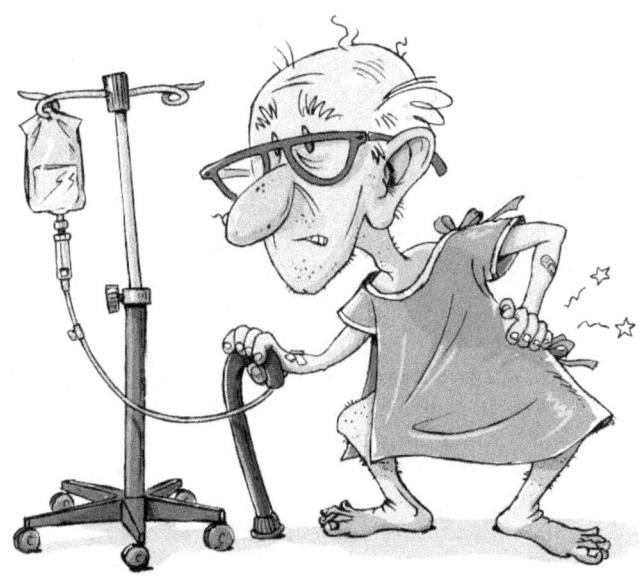

The geriatric population needs special care due to their multiple comorbidities.

Special considerations:

- **Always assess:** mental status, living situation (family/ alone/nursing home/personnal care), functional capacity, handling finances, primary physician follow up adherence, accuracy in taking meds (or maybe forget doses?), Code status, ride on discharge, & ability to eat/drink (any special diet?).
- **Obtaining hx** can be difficult because of dementia, hearing loss, anxiety, confusion, stroke/aphasia→ask closed ended yes/no answer questions.
- **Obtain permission** (if possible) & hx from caregiver & family members, nursing home staff, personal care home staff
- **Meds review**: Many pts will NOT know their meds & /or doses; ask family members or contact pharmacy where they get Tx filled. Cr Clearance ↓ w/ age; many renally eliminated meds have to be dose adjusted.

Attention: Ask about OTC drugs & stop meds can cause side effects like AMS w/ Fluoroquinolone, Diphenhydramine or even benzodiazepines (paroxysmuse effect)

- **Functional Inquiry:**
  BADLs- Basic Activities of Daily Living (aka ADLs, personal self-care): toileting, bathing, grooming, feeding, ambulation- independently or w/ assistance, or total dependence on others
  IADLs- Instrumental Activities of Daily Living (using tools & instruments): laundry, shopping, accounting, driving, housekeeping, & meds
- **Living situation:** Alone/w/ family/nursing home/personal care home/homeless.

- **Power of attorney:** legal document that allows the pt to designate someone else to perform certain duties on their behalf. Can be written to become effective if clinical condition changes & they become incapacitated
- **Advance Directive:** choice on what life-saving Tx they choose to receive when their heart stops beating or they stop breathing
- Consider assessing **code status** while the pt can make decisions in order to respect the pt's wishes in case of acute health deterioration occurs. DNR=do NOT resuscitate, DNI= do NOT intubate
- **Beers Criteria**: is a tool, which can be used to avoid inappropriate meds use in older adults from the American Geriatrics Society in order to improve meds safety in older adults (**available online**).

38. Palliative/supportive care & hospice care

Sometimes, part of the management is NOT curative & we treat pts supportively w/ palliative care for a period of time until they move to in/out pt hospice, as is the case w/ some common incurable terminal cases. As doctors, we need to be w/ the pts all the way down the road & make them as comfortable as possible.

Examples of common palliative care cases w/ management:

- **Sickle cell disease pain**: from recurrent vaso-occlusions due to deoxygenated Hgb polymerization. Use Tylenol & NSAIDS (ibuprofen, naproxen, & ketorolac) for mild to moderate pain. For severe pain, use opioids like Percocet, dilaudid, morphine, methadone, meperidine, or long acting opioids like MS Contin or fentanyl patches.
  PCA is another option for in pt management (you can order basal & PRN pain meds). Switch to PO pain meds if appropriate when anticipating a discharge in the next 24 hrs. Check kidney function for NSAIDs, & exclude pain emergencies like Acute Chest Syndrome (ACS) & priapism (Tx is plasmapheresis).
- **Cancer** (mostly managed by Heme/Onc): early detection of the cancer is essential for curativeTx (T1 or T2 w/ N0M0 for solid tumors). CT scans, PET scans, & bone scans can play a role in staging & prognosis. Delivering the diagnosis w/ sympathy & support is part of Tx.
- **Malignant hypercalcemia**: can sometimes be the 1st indication of malignancy (PTH should be suppressed or inappropriately normal). It can present asymptomatically or w/ nonspecific Sx like dehydration & confusion. **Tx:** Hydration w/

mostly normal saline (considerlasix), PO or IV bisphosphonates, & steroids.

- **SIADH:** Causes euvolemic hyponatremia. Hypo or hypervolemic hyponatremia suggests other causes for ↓ Na^+ besides SIADH such as either a CNS process like metastasis or small cell lung cancer. Tx: only Symptomatic pts (like those w/ change in baseline neurologic status) w/ hypertonic solutions like 3% NS. Caution against rapid correction as it can cause demyelinating disorder. Discontinuation of some drugs, such as HCTZ, could cause SIADH. Consider fluid restriction for chronic hyponatremia >48 hrs (target UOP 500cc daily).
- **Nausea & vomiting:** common Sx & common meds side effect. Tx: zofran, phenergan or reglan. You can use them together for refractory Sx. Consider NG tube if meds alone are NOT effective.
- **Constipation:** r/o small bowel obstruction (no air-fluid levels on abdomen xray), acute abdomen (rigidity, guarding & rebound tenderness), & mechanical obstruction as in colon cancer as the Tx for these may be surgical. Tx: fibers, Miralax, milk of Mg, lactulose, senna & golytely
- **Stents:** easy & fast procedure can be used in the case of pancreatic head cancer, superior vena cava syndrome, esophagus/gastric cancer w/ GI obstruction effect or any stenosis for temporary relief.
- **Anorexia:** from cancer, an end stage diseases like ESRD, COPD, & CHF, or meds such as chemotherapy. It can cause cachexia. Tx: Megestrol (long term), steroids (short term, <8weeks), exercise, & optimization of nutrition intake (if possible).
- **Pleural effusion:** especially malignant effusion, treat only if Symptomatic. Tx: Thoracentesis (assess for relief of Sx after intervention & rate

of re-accumulation), chest tube (pleurex tube), &
pleurodesis (last resort). Sometimes it is hard to
control.
- **Ascites:** especially associated w/ malignant &
  hepatic cirrhosis. Tx: sprinolactone,
  paracentesis, consider TIPS (transjugular
  intrahepatic portosystemic shunt), & weigh the
  risk of hepatoencephalopathy in cirrhosis.

Attention: to dementia pts especially under hospice when
they canNOT express pain as the signs of pain is grins &
moaning w/ hands clinching & vitals changing (HTN &
tachycardia)

- **Calculate scores** to assess the **severity** of the
  disease like: MELD for liver cirrhosis (& help in
  assessment of transplant). Other commonly
  used scores are: CHADS2 for a fib & the need
  for anticoagx, Ranson criteria for pancreatitis, &
  Duke Criteria for endocarditis diagnosis.

Special Considerations:

Discuss DNR/DNI early in the process when the pt is
oriented & can still make decisions so that we may
respect the pt's wishes.
After the pt, Power of Attorney (POA) is the next in line
to make a decision.
If NOT available, next of kin has the right to make
decisions.

Attention: DNR/DNI means do NOT resuscitate/intubate & does
NOT mean "do NOT treat." A lot of pts like to be DNR but also
they want everything to be done if they got sick (very reasonable
as they did NOT decline Tx w/ the DNR/DNI). Some pts will
maybe specify limited intervention w/ the DNR/DNI like no ICU
level of care, no vasopressors, no surgeries, & so forth. Talk w/
the pt or the decision maker about how aggressive they wish their
medical intervention to be.

Qualification for hospice:
- Any pt with life expectancy <6 months; whatever the disease is
- Certain invasive cancer pts (fail or decline Tx)
- End stage CHF (NYHA stage IV inspite of maximizing medical TX)
- Severe COPD (resting SOB inspite of breathing Tx & home O_2)
- End stage liver cirrhosis/disease (symptomatic w/max Tx, refractory ascites, ↓ albumin/↑ INR or hepatoencephalopathy & NOT candidate for transplant for like: active EtOH abuse)
- CVA/dementia with general declining
- ESRD on HD w/ uremia Sx (or plan to stop dialysis due to access difficulties).

Family meetings: with pt's family who have serious illness or maybe terminal is very helpful to put the medical team, the pt & the family on "the same page" by discussing the prognosis & the Tx options. Such meetings offer the pt support & giving them the data & the option for proceeding or maybe declining Tx as appropriate. Lack of communication w/ families may lead to disappointments & maybe unnecessary legal problems.

Pronouncing death: Examine the pt by checking for the absence of heartbeats & breathing sounds for almost a minute & the absence of brain stem reflexes such as the gag & corneal reflexes. Checking the heart monitor is an easier way to monitor cardiac activity although it can be present even if the pt is dead in case of a pacemaker. Pronounce the time of death, offer the family help, & proceed w/ the paper work.

Know the reason of death (or what you think is the most probable reason, sometimes there are multiple). Ask the family about autopsy, organ donation, & funeral home arrangements, as this information will be needed for the paper work.

Brain death: simply means that there is no any brain activity either cortical (absence to purposeful movement like no withdrawal to pain or absence of normal vestibule-ocular reflexes or brain stem (like spontaneous breathing & corneal/papillary light/gag reflex) activity. Pt will be ventilator dependent, basically, but the heart is the only thing working. The legal criteria are more complicated & it is better to be done by neurologist.

Miscellaneous

39. Diabetes mellitus (DM)

Diabetes Mellitus (DM) is a common metabolic disturbance seen in U. S adults & occurs due to a defect in insulin secretion, action, or both. Around 11% of the U. S population >20 years old is affected. Around 90% of those cases belong to the type II category.

Classification: The majority of cases can be classified into one of two categories: type I (<10%) & type II (>90%). Other specific types of DM exist related to certain genetic defects, drugs, endocrinopathies, & other syndromes. Also, DM related to pregnancy is known as gestational diabetes mellitus (resolved after delivery, recurrent in subsequent gestations, & can become overt DM).

Diagnosis: suggested by any of the following criteria:
1. Plasma glucose > 126 mg/dl after an overnight fast (should be confirmed w/ a repeat test). Fasting glucose level between 100-125 mg/dl indicates Impaired Fasting Glucose (IFG).
2. Random glucose level > 200 mg/dl plus Sx of diabetes mellitus (polyuria, polydipsia, fatigue, weight loss). Values of 140-199 mg/dl indicate Impaired Glucose Tolerance (IGT).
3. PO glucose tolerance test, which shows a glucose level > 200 mg/dl 2 hrs after administration of a 75 gm glucose load.
4. HgbA1c>6. 5% (needs to be confirmed w/ any of the above).

Management: Glycemic control & management of other atherosclerosis risk factors like HTN (JNC-8 guidelines, target has changed to BP <140/90), HLD (LDL goal is <100 mg/dl), smoking, & monitor for diabetic end organ damage such as retinopathy & glomerulopathy (by early referral to ophthalmology, w/ in 10 years for type I & on the time of diagnoses for type II, & referral to nephrology in CKD stage III). Fasting CBG should be between 70 to 130 mg/dl & postprandial CBG should be targeted to <180 mg/dl w/ Hgb A1c < 7%. For in pt (especially critically ill pts) target CBG should NOT be strictly controlled → okay <180 to avoid hypoglycemia. Consider more strict A1c control (<5.5%) in CF & pregnant pts.

DM Type I: Type I requires lifelong insulin replacement. The sooner DM II is diagnosed, the more insulin secreting beta cells will be saved from destruction & the easier DM will be managed.

Type of insulin	Onset of action (hrs)	Peak effect (hrs)	Effect duration (hrs)
Rapid acting			
Lispro/Aspart/Glulisine	<15min	≈1	3-5
Regular (draw 1st in syringe if mixed w/ NPH)	≈1	2-4	6-8
Intermediate acting			
NPH (only one cloudy, rest clear)	≈1.5	6-8	12-16
Long acting			
Glargine	1-2	0	Up to 24
Levemir/Detemir	1-2	0	Up to 24

Usually, in an average pt, total daily dose (TDD) of insulin is calculated by the following formula: 0.2-0.8 units/kg per day (0. 2 units/kg is usually started in a newly diagnosed/insulin naive pt). About 50% of the dose is usually basal insulin (intermediate or long-acting insulin, either NPH twice daily or detemir/glargine once daily), & the rest can be divided to three times/day before meals (or even twice depending on the compliance).

Two of the most commonly used regimens are:

1. **NPH & regular (2-3 injections/day):** Calculate Total Daily Dose TDD as per 0.4-0.8 units/kg. Divide it ½ & ½ OR 2/3rd & 1/3rd in morning & evening, depending on the biggest meal in the day. Divide the morning dose administered w/ breakfast into 2/3rd NPH & 1/3rd regular.

    Divide the evening dose into ½ NPH (to be administered at bedtime) & ½ regular (to be administered w/ evening meal). Then, calculate the correction factor by the following formula: 1700 divided by the TDD.
    This means that 1 unit of insulin will bring down the glucose by approximately x mg (x-correction factor, try to make the numbers easy to calculate like 50, 60, etc.). **Correction factor calculation is time consuming & can be avoided safely most of the time.**

    This regimen is also the cheapest available on the market. It is a good regimen for non-insured, newly diagnosed DM, & non-compliant pts as it needs fewer sticks.
    NPH & regular insulin can be prescribed also as a pre-mixed combination of 70% NPH/30% regular regimen (commonly known as 70/30) & it can be given twice daily (before breakfast & lunch or lunch & dinner, depends on the two largest meals)

2. **Glargine & aspart/lispro/regular (four times a day regimen):** Usually 50% of TDD is administered as long-acting glargine at night, & the remaining dose is divided into 3 times a day as rapid acting insulin given w/ meals.

    Supplemental sliding scale SSS can be added to the scheduled doses for better DM control (increase the scheduled insulin dose according to the previous day requirement from the SSS).

CBGs should be monitored both as an in pt & as an out pt at least 3-4 times/day (2 times is acceptable for out pt). Monitoring should include fasting CBG pre-breakfast & random post-prandial checks (writing them in a log can help in adjusting insulin doses).

Type II DM: Initial therapy is w/ PO agents. **Metformin** is commonly used as it has an added benefit of reducing obesity (↓ mortality as well). Also, it does NOT cause hypoglycemia (adverse reactions: N/V, & diarrhea). However, it should be used w/ caution in pts w/ renal disease (avoid in CKDIII or more as it could cause lactic acidosis). Sulfonylureas (SFU) such as glipizide, glyburide, & glimepiride are also used commonly.

Other non-SFU analogues such as nateglinide & repaglinide are rarely used. Other options include alpha-glucosidase inhibitor acarbose, thiazolidinediones such as rosiglitazone or pioglitazone (can cause fluid retention & should thus be used w/ caution in cardiac or renal disease), dipeptidyl peptidase-4 inhibitors sitagliptin & saxagliptin, bile acid sequestrant colesevelam, & glucagon-like peptide agonists such as exenatide. Eventually, type II DM pts end up needing insulin, which should be started as discussed above.

Diabetic ketoacidosis:
DKA occurs in up to 5% of pts w/ type I DM & can rarely occur in type II DM as well. It is often precipitated due to interruption of insulin dose when the pt feels sick. Precipitating factors could be a UTI, PNA, sepsis, MI, or trauma.
Usually include polyuria, polydipsia, N/V, abdominal pain, & signs of dehydration. Labs will show an elevated anion gap metabolic acidosis, elevated CBGs (however DKA can also rarely occur w/ normal CBGs), & electrolyte abnormalities.

Management:
Should include **fluid replacement therapy & insulin.** Fluid replacement therapy is extremely important & should be started w/o delay. There is a fluid deficit of several liters, which should be replaced w/ normal saline boluses until vital signs stabilize & urine output is established.

After initial boluses, free water deficit is replaced w/ maintenance fluids (either normal saline or 0. 45% saline at 150–500 ml/hr for severe hypernatremia; always remember to correct Na for CBG).
Insulin therapy is usually started w/ initial fluid replacement. A bolus of regular insulin at 0.1 units/kg is given as soon as possible. Then, an insulin drip at 0.1 units/kg/hr is started. CBG should be lowered gradually at a rate of 50-75 mg/dl/hr (excess rapid correction>100 mg/dl/hr can lead to osmotic encephalopathy).

BMP & CBGs need to be monitored every 2 hrs. Once CBG reaches 250 mg/dL, fluids should be changed to dextrose (5%) in 0. 45% saline to prevent dangerous hypoglycemia.

Insulin drip is continued until anion gap closes & pt has clinically improved. Subcutaneous insulin is usually started once pt starts eating. Always remember to continue the insulin drip for an hr after administration of subcutaneous insulin as it takes time to take effect.

Potassium: K deficit should always be anticipated, even if initial BMP shows normal K, as insulin administration can cause shift of K intracellularly. K should be routinely added to IV fluids at a rate of 10-20 meq/hr except in pts w/ hyperkalemia (>6 mmol/hr), renal failure, or oliguria. Bicarbonate, phosphate, & Mg rarely need to be replaced.

Bicarbonate: therapy in DKA is indicated only if pH <7. 1, shock/coma, plasma bicarbonate <5, acidosis-induced cardiorespiratory dysfunction, or severe hyperkalemia. When discharging pts w/ DKA, always remember to provide DM education to prevent further episodes.

Hyperosmolar non-ketotic syndrome (HONK):

Commonly seen in type II DM. It is very similar to DKA w/ some difference. HONK is typically more insidious in onset w/ dehydration (due to diuresis effect of the very high blood glucose) & some neurological deficits. No or mild ketoacidosis in HONK (PH >7.30 & HCO3 >15) compared to DKA (anion gab metabolic acidosis) due to the presence of insulin in the former (prevent lipolysis). **Tx:** same as DKA; especially **IV hydration**.

Hypoglycemia:

Common in the in pt setting & is often iatrogenic or caused by inadequate PO intake.

Management:

For conscious pts, orange juice, candy bars, fruits, & crackers can be given immediately (or Glucose tablets). IV dextrose should be used for pts w/ AMS. Initial bolus of 20 to 50 mL of 50% dextrose followed by an infusion D5W should be administered w/o delay.

Glucagon 1 mg IM/SC can be administered for those who are unable to take PO or who do NOT have IV access (or pts w/ "bad veins" & hard to get IV access on).

Complications of diabetes:

Long-term complications are divided into microvascular & macrovascular. Microvascular include diabetic retinopathy (usually the 1st one to occur), nephropathy, & neuropathy. Coronary artery disease & peripheral vascular disease are some of the macrovascular complications.

> **Attention**: Tight CBG control (A1c <6.5-7%)→ reduce microvascular complications w/ minimal to no benefit for macrovascular complications (so pts w/ CVA, PAD or CAD may target A1c 7-8, especially w/ hx of hypoglycemia). Young pts → A1c <6.5-7%.

Routine screening: Pts w/ newly diagnosed type II DM should get an ophthalmology referral (yearly) to screen for diabetic retinopathy (possible laser Tx for non/proliferative retinopathy or "leaky vessels" to prevent blindness). For type I DM, it is usually recommended 5 years after diagnosis. Urine microalbumin (yearly), lipid panel, neurological exam & detailed foot exam should be done in yearly basis or more often (PRN).

Special considerations:
- **ACE inhibitors or ARBs are recommended** as 1st line for HTN w/ DM as they are known to prevent renal complications.
- **Standard insulin concentration is 100 units/mL (U-100).** Rarely, a highly concentrated form of insulin U-500 (500 units/mL) is used (when you need a very high dose of U-100 like 100s)
- **Diabetes mellitus in hospitalized pts:** Numerous studies have been done on glycemic control in hospitalized pts. The generally accepted target is 140 for floor pts & 180 for ICU pts (or critically ill pts). Avoidance of hypoglycemia should be a priority in both ICU & non-ICU pts.
- **In general: Insulin should be started for all DM type I & DM type II if oral meds failed** to control A1c (<6.5 - 7%). Consider starting insulin for DM type II if A1c is very high on the initial presentation (like >10%) due to the fact that oral

meds ↓ A1c around 1% per one med (usually you can NOT use more than 3 oral meds). Certain compliant pts can still control their A1c with diet, exercise & oral meds even if A1c is >10 on the presentation.

- **Supplemental insulin (less preferred term is sliding scale insulin):** is commonly used in addition to the scheduled dose for in pt to better control CBG. For optimal DM management, scheduled doses should be adjusted in a daily bases (at AM) according to the previous day supplemental insulin doses (if the pt expected to have the same calorie intake). So if pt is scheduled for 5 U aspart before dinner & he/she took 2 U after dinner on the supplemental scale → give 7 U aspart instead of 5 U the next evening.

- **Hypoglycemia:** usually when CBG <50-60.
  Sx: AMS (even coma) and/or sympathetic nervous system stimulation (palpitation, sweating, & anxiety).
  Etiology: diabetics w/ insulin over dosing, skipping meals, oral diabetes meds (especially in setting of AKI or CKD), sepsis, adrenal insufficiency, EtOH or exercise (w/o ↓ insulin dose).
  Management: check A1c, cortisol, TSH, UDS, possible infx, & C peptide (exogenous insulin?). Consider glucose tolerance test, review meds (especially new ones) & prediabetes (in DMII when insulin resistance ↑ →reactive hypoglycemia from ↑ insulin secretion after meals →Tx w/ metformin!). Tx w/ PO sugary fluid, IV dextrose (amp of D50% or drip D5/D10).

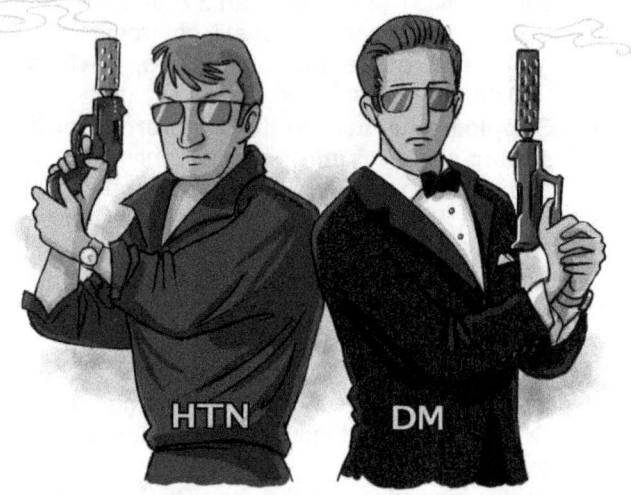

"THE SILENT KILLERS"

HTN & DM are the "silent killers" & may NOT cause
symptoms. Treat & follow the numbers as appropriate.

40. Anticoagulation

Various drugs are used for anticoagx, known as 'blood thinners' in layman terminology. There are different indications & guidelines for each of them & therefore, each of them will be discussed separately.

Heparin:

Mechanism of action: activates anti-thrombin III, which inactivates clotting enzymes, such as thrombin & Factor Xa. Two major formulations of heparin are unfractionated heparin (UFH) & low-molecular weight heparin (LMWH). LMWH mainly acts by inactivating factor Xa.

Uses: Heparin & its other formulations are used for treating venous thromboembolism (VTE), which includes both deep vein thrombosis (DVT) & pulm embolism. Guidelines recommend treating any episode of VTE w/ 4-5 days of either UFH heparin (IV heparin drip) or LMWH like Enoxaparin (subcutaneous injection), while "bridging" w/ Coumadin to maintain therapeutic INR for at least 2 days before discharge.
For UFH (IV drip), there is a weight-based heparin dosing protocol (nurses usually manage it by a protocol). Therefore, the pt has to be admitted to the hospital. LMWH also has a weight-based dosing. However, it is a subcutaneous injection & so pts can be discharged on it.

LMWH is contraindicated in pts w/ renal insufficiency: avoid in ESR & requires dose adjustments in pts w/ eGFR <30 (once daily instead of twice daily dosing). Heparin (subcutaneous) & LMWH (at lower doses) are also used as prophylaxis to prevent episodes of VTE in immobilized pts, including pts lying in hospital beds for long periods of time.

Adverse effects: Heparin-induced thrombocytopenia (HIT) can develop w/ any dose or type of heparin, & is of two types. Type 1 is a non-immune mediated process where the decline in platelet count is w/ in the first 24-48 hrs, & does NOT require stopping heparin. Type 2 is an immune-mediated process where the decline in platelet count occurs between 5-14 days, & requires stopping all forms of heparin. Type 2 may require Tx w/ argatroban due to high risk of associated arterial or venous thrombosis. Other adverse effects include hyperkalemia & osteoporosis.

Warfarin:

Mechanism of action: acts by inhibiting vitamin-K dependent pro-coagulant factors, namely factors II, VII, IX, X & anti-coagulant factors, protein C & S synthesized by the liver. It takes about 5 days to achieve full anti-coagulant effect. Initially, due to rapid depletion of Protein C before the other pro-coagulant factors, there is a risk of hypercoagulability & warfarin-induced skin necrosis. Therefore, heparin therapy should be used in the first 2-3days of anticoagx, along w/ Coumadin (bridging therapy). When beginning Warfarin, INR needs to be checked w/ in the first week to make dosage adjustments, then carefully monitored monthly. Also, you have to consider the dangers of using Warfarin in an elderly pt at risk for falls (weigh risks & benefits w/ the pt or his/her family).

Uses:

Tx of VTE: After about 5 days of heparin, an episode of DVT or pulm embolism requires long-term Tx w/ an PO anti-coagulant for several months. Duration depends on risk of recurrent VTE & bleeding – first episode of VTE w/ reversible factors such as immobilization due to trauma, surgery, PO contraceptive pills, & long-duration air travel requires Tx for 3 months. Pts w/ cancer should receive anticoagx until cancer resolves. Pts w/ inherited hypercoagulable states, such as Factor V Leiden, or Protein C, S or ATIII deficiencies usually require Tx for over 6 months. If a pt has recurrent idiopathic VTE, they require anticoagx for life unless contraindications such hemorrhage develops.

Anticoagx for artificial heart valves: Target INR depends on the type of heart valve used. For any tissue valve at any location, target INR is between 2-3 for 3 months & then lifelong ASA. If a mechanical (metal) valve is placed, pt will mostly need lifelong Coumadin (depends on the valve location mitral/aortic & the type St. Jude's or others).

Anticoagx for a fib: People w/ A fib are at an ↑ risk for stroke. A CHADS2 score is a simple pneumonic to help assess the risk of stroke in a pt w/ non-rheumatic a fib. CHADS2 stands for **Congestive** heart Failure (1 point), **HTN** (1 point), **A**ge ≥75 years (1 point), **D**iabetes mellitus (1 point), & prior hx of **S**troke or TIA (**2** points, hence the 2 by the S). Generally, a score of 2 or above is considered a strong indication for anticoagx.

CHA2DS2VASc scoring system is more accurate tool **(use if CHADS2 score is 0 or 1)** to assess the need for anticoagx (especially elderly women). It stands for CHF (1 point), HTN (1 point), Age ≥ 75 (2 points), DM (1 point), Stroke (2 points), Vascular disease (1 point), Age 65-74 (1 point), Sex (Sex category w/ 1 point if female). Female w/ a score of ≥ 2 needs to be considered for long-term anticoagx (or male ≥ 1).

How to reverse a high INR from Coumadin overdose: For asymptomatic minor INR elevations (INR <5), no intervention is needed other than holding Coumadin & then restarting it at a lower dose once INR is in target range. For an INR between 5-9 (w/o bleeding), hold all anti-thrombotic therapy, & repeat INR again the next day. If the INR is still rising or there is a high risk of bleeding, give vitamin K PO (usually, a low dose such as 1mg is preferred).

If the **INR is >9 (w/o bleeding),** give vitamin K (2-10 mg PO) & repeat the INR in 24-28 hrs. Repeat the vitamin K dose as needed (needs hours to days to work).

If there is a **minor bleed w/ any INR level**, vitamin K 1-5 mg PO or IV must be given. Recheck INR in 24 hrs & if it still NOT controlled, repeat the vitamin K dosage. If bleeding still persists after repeat vitamin K, it must be treated as a major bleed.

Any **major bleeding** for a pt on Coumadin should be treated w/ vitamin K IV 10 mg over 10-20 minutes & FFP (rechecked INR in 6-12 hrs) & continue vitamin K & FFP until bleeding has stopped. Surgical intervention to stop the bleeding may also be considered.

Anticoagx after coronary artery stenting: Current guidelines recommend anticoagx w/ dual anti-platelet therapy (DAPT), which includes ASA w/ either clopidogrel (most commonly used) or others such as prasugrel, ticagrelor, or ticlopidine. Duration of therapy for both drug-eluting stents (DES) & bare metal stents (BMS) is 12 months. Minimum duration of uninterrupted therapy is 4 weeks for BMS, & 6 months for DES (every effort to continue therapy should be made prior to stopping at this early duration). Sometimes for repeated stenting & extensive CAD, Plavix & ASA should be considered for life if NOT contraindicated (e.g., tendency to bleed)

Novel PO anticoagulants: Dabigatran (Pradaxa), apixaban (Eliquis), & rivaroxaban (Xarelto) are novel PO anticoagulants that can be used as alternatives to warfarin in certain circumstances, such as in non-valvular a fib stroke prevention. These have an advantage in that there is no need to monitor INR, & there is ↓ risk of bleeding, especially w/ apixaban & rivaroxaban. However, in the event of a major bleed, there are still no reversal agents for these new agents, as is the case w/ warfarin. They are associated w/ ↓ risk of major bleeding episodes such as intra-cranial bleeds, but have high risk of GI bleeds. Usually they are expensive & some insurance companies do NOT cover them.

Special consideration:

- **Heparin IV drip is preferred for critically ill pts or those expected to have surgical intervention** (e.g., CABG or heart catheterization) due to the quick wash off period (short half-life; 4-6hours). LMWH has longer half-life of 12-24 hrs. So "bridging" from oral anticoagx like warfarin to IV heparin drip is necessary by holding the warfarin & monitoring INR daily. Start heparin drip when INR is subtherapeutic (<2 or 2.5).

Attention: Do NOT stop heparin drip unless the procedure/surgery is confirmed & resume heparin ASAP simultaneously w/ warfarin until INR is therapeutic. Successful "bridging" is important especially for pts with mechanical valves.

- **Pts on anticoagx (like warfarin) who presented w/ bleeding (usually from GI tract):** INR should be checked & may be reversed as indicated above, considering the INR level & severity of the bleed. Consider resuming warfarin after Tx (e.g., clipping or cauterizing a bleeding source EGD & colonoscopy) & you may need to discuss risk & benefits of resuming anticoagx meds w/ the pt in case of recurrence.
- **Facts about Plavix:**
  A. Need to be stopped five days before any non-emergent surgery (e.g., CABG) to be "washed out" & ↓ the bleeding risk.
  B. Hold off giving plavix at the time of chest pain presentation for pts who may need CABG after the heart cath (like elderly w/ DM or ESRD on HD). Plavix can be given at the time of the heart cath if stent/s are indicated.

C. All efforts should be made to keep Plavix for at least 6months s/p DES & 6weeks s/p BMS to prevent in-stent stenosis (try to postpone any elective surgeries until after these dates).

- **Triple oral antithrombotic therapy (TOAT)** is needed sometimes for cardiovascular disease. It means the concomitant use of dual antiplatelet therapy (DAPT) w/ aspirin & ADP platelet receptor blocker like Plavix or Effient (as s/p DUS) & oral anticoagulation (OAC) like after A fib diagnosis w/ high CHADS2 score ($\geq$ 2). All efforts should be made to stop any of them when they are NOT indicated anymore due to the high bleeding risk (stop plavix after 1 yr of DUS). INR should be monitored more frequently (target INR is different in TOAT, metal valve: 2. 5-3, a fib: 2-2. 5).

- **Screening for thrombophilia & malignancy following a first episode of unprovoked venothrombotic event (VTE) is controversial.** Limited cancer screening is acceptable for the 1stepisode of idiopathic VTE (i.e., no CT/PET scans) with a clinical evaluation (focused malignancy hx like weight loss, $\downarrow$ appetite, SOB, constipation or hematuria), basic laboratory testing (like CBC, CMP, & ESR), age-appropriate cancer screening (like mammogram, & colonoscopy as indicated) & CXR (& following the abnormal results w/ full work up). More extensive cancer screening strategies are NOT justified in this population but may be warranted for higher cancer risk pts (like recurrent VTE despite anticoagx & hepatic or portal vein thrombosis).

  If you decided to go with the extensive thrombophilia work up (like after the 2nd VTE), **postpone the tests for few weeks** (mostly as an out pt) after the even as the clotting even & the anticoagx meds will affect the tests results. Factor V Leiden, prothrombin gene mutation, antiphospholipid antibodies, factor C & S deficiency are prothrombogenic factors. Surgery (especially orthopedics), pregnancy, oral contraceptives, immobilization, CHF, & central lines are common acquired etiology as well.

- **Prophylactic anticoagulation:** is very important to prevent DVT/PE in certain populations in addition to the in pt DVT prophylaxis (heparin 5000 u TID or LMWH like Daltiparin –better- or Lovenox). Pts w/ fractures, immobile, or cancer may need 3-6 months of lovenox (preferred for oncology pts) or oral anticoagx agents. Clinical trials support that prophylaxis & showing good mortality benefits but guidelines is still NOT totally supporting it, yet (consult hematology PRN). IVC filter is a controversial option to prevent PE (commonly it is indicated to prevent 2nd PE in pts with known DVT who had 1st PE & failed anticoagx).

41. Anemia

Anemia is defined as Hgb<14 for male & <12 for a female. Caused by either a ↓ in RBC production, or an↑ in destruction (hemolysis) or loss (bleeding).

Acute RBC loss from a bleed manifests as pallor, fatigue, dyspnea on exertion, dizziness, syncope, & angina (if they have concomitant CAD).

Chronic anemia has fewer Sx because the body has become accustomed to it. However, even if it is a chronic anemia, pt will usually be Symptomatic if the Hgb<7.

The reticulocyte index (different than the reticulocyte count) is an indicator for the bone marrow's response to ↓ RBCs. If the RI<2%, this indicates bone marrow response is poor & there is hypoproliferation of RBCs. If RI >2%, the bone marrow is responding appropriately to RBC loss or destruction.
In general, it is important to know if the bone marrow has adequate response to know what you are dealing w/ Is it hemolysis or bleeding loss? (Elevated RI, i. e the BM is working) or production problem (↓ RI like Leukemias or B12 deficiency).

Classification:
a. **Microcytic anemia (**MCV <80):
Iron deficiency anemia: This is the most common cause found in adults.

Etiology: chronic GI bleeding (gastritis, GI ulcers, & undiagnosed malignancy), ↑ demand, (e.g. pregnancy), ↓ supply (malnutrition & abnormal absorption in the GI tract, such as in celiac or Crohn's disease).

Work up: Order iron studies including iron, TIBC, & ferritin. In iron deficiency anemia, iron & ferritin should be low, & TIBC should be high. If the ferritin is <15, it greatly indicates iron deficiency anemia. If it is >200, it excludes iron deficiency as the cause of the anemia.

Management: Ferrous sulfate PO (could cause GI upset, black stool & constipation) or IV iron if indicated. Indications for IV iron include intolerance to PO, or a need for high dose iron, such as in an ongoing bleed. Consideration: do NOT treat microcytic anemia w/ iron unless it is indicated, due to the possibility of missing a colon cancer as a reason of anemia.

b. **Macrocytic anemia** (MCV>100):

Folate deficiency:
Etiology (can occur after a few months of deficiency): malnutrition, high demand (hemolysis, pregnancy/lactation), EtOH & poor diet, elderly, dialysis pts, & pts taking anti-folic acid meds, such as methotrexate.

B12 deficiency:
Etiology (needs to be present for greater than 3years to occur): partial or total gastrectomy, pernicious anemia, pancreatic insufficiency, malnutrition (alcoholics, vegans), & bacterial overgrowth.

Diagnosis is similar for B12 & folate deficiency by: CBC showing macrocytic anemia, a ↓ reticulocyte count, blood smear w/ hypersegmented neutrophils present, high LDH & indirect bilirubin (reflecting ineffective erythropoiesis), & ↓ serum B12 & folate.
The difference between folate & B12 deficiency: In B12 deficiency, methylmalonic acid (MMA) & homocysteine (HCY) are elevated, & peripheral neuropathy can be present from subacute combined degeneration along w/ hypersegmented PMNs in peripheral blood smear. In folic acid deficiency, only homocysteine is elevated & there are no neurological findings.

Management: Vitamin replacement.

Special consideration:

- **Consider bone marrow aspiration/biopsy** if B12/folate is normal & exclude alcoholism to r/o MDS & aplastic anemia.
- **Infective Erythropoiesis:** happens in B12 or folate deficiency when the premature blood cells hemolyze in the BM due to the need for these vitamins for maturation process/DNA synthesis & that gives an intravascular hemolysis picture w/ elevated LDH, ↓ haptoglobin, & elevated indirect bilirubin.
- **Reticulocytosis starts in one week of therapy,** & Hgb rises in 6-8 weeks. K can become depleted due to hematopoiesis; & therefore, may need to be replenished. A common cause of incomplete response to therapy is coexisting iron deficiency.
- **Prophylactic replacement** w/ ↓ doses for pregnancy, lactation, & hemolytic states should be considered, especially for folic acid as the stores are ↓ & can be depleted faster.

c. **Normocytic anemia** (MCV 80-100):
Anemia of chronic disease (including CKD/ESRD):
Etiology: autoimmune disorder, chronic infx, cancer, or HIV pts.
Work up: no specific tests are diagnostic, but order iron studies. Ferritin should be high, as it is an inflammatory marker; however, it can be normal. Iron can be low or normal. TIBC will be low (or normal). Soluble transferrin receptor is normal (but high in iron deficiency).

Acute bleeding (very common):
Acute bleeding will cause a normocytic anemia while chronic bleeding (usually from GI loss) will cause iron stores depletion & microcytic anemia. Bleeding could be from GI tract (ulcers, diverticulosis, hemorrhoids, etc.) or external from trauma for instance. Assess the severity from the vitals, as tachycardia indicates a loss of at least

10% of the blood volume, orthostatic HoTN (>20 mmHg ↓ in SBP or >10 ↑ in heart rate when standing compared to sitting) indicates>20% loss, while shock (HoTN w/ organ failure) may indicate>30% loss. Hgb & hematocrit are poor indicators for the amount of blood loss in the case of acute bleeding, as it needs time for the concentration to go down.

Management: 2 large bore (14-16 gauge) IV caths need to be in place for fluid resuscitation. Fluid resuscitation w/ normal saline, blood transfusion, or reverse coagulopathy (by FFP or vitamin K as indicated) can be considered.
Triage to the ICU if the pt is still hypotensive for vasopressors to keep mean arterial pressure MAP>65 to prevent organs ischemia. Consider surgical evaluation for possible ongoing bleeding (intrathoracic/abdomen & in the thighs). Always place pressure on overt superficial bleeding.

Special consideration:
- **Coexisting iron deficiency is common** & ferritin can be ↓. Positive response to PO iron in a few weeks can be diagnostic.
- **ESRD pts can have functional iron deficiency** even if ferritin >500. Erythropoietin (Epo) is only helpful if it is ↓ (<500 mU/mL), & is NOT indicated in anemia of chronic disease w/ normal erythropoietin levels. Epo level can be obtained in a simple blood test.
- **A GI bleed is usually obvious** due to the stimulant effect of the blood in the intestines. Examine the thighs periodically (consider CT scan to confirm bleeding) if you suspect bleeding for any reason in that area due to hip fractures, trauma, or recent intervention like post cardiac cath w/ femoral access or femoral dialysis cath. These areas can contain 1-2 liters of blood & show minimal changes.

Hemolysis:

Sickle cell disease: When HgbS becomes deoxygenated, it polymerizes & then the RBC sickles, which causes ↓ RBC deformability & leads to hemolysis & occlusion. A pt can present w/ the hemolysis picture, including jaundice, as well as vascular occlusion. The most common presentation is acute painful episodes or sickle cell pain crisis, which manifests as generalized pain mostly in long bones, back, chest & the abdomen. Precipitating factors include dehydration, infx, stress, EtOH use, & weather. However, the majority of cases have no identifiable trigger. Acute chest syndrome (CP, ↓ O_2 saturation & infiltration on CXR) & priapism are an indication for exchange transfusion.

Work up: hemolysis labs. Get blood smear & Hgb electrophoresis if the pt is NOT diagnosed already (as it can determine the presence of any hemoglobinopathies like SCD & thalassemia, etc).

Tx:

Acutely: Hydration (3-4L/day), pain control (morphine or a dilaudid PCA pump), antipyretics, & empiric abx (after blood/urine/sputum culture along w/ urinalysis & CXR)

> **Chronically:** Hydroxyurea, which ↑Hgb F & ↓Sx. Folic acid is used because depletion of folic acid can make the anemia worse, & they are in constant turnover w/ sickle cell disease. These pts need to stay hydrated & avoid hypoxia. The only curative option is a bone marrow transplant, & it is usually a last option.

> **Attention:** Immunizations are important in sickle cell pts, including Pneumovax & the meningococcal vaccine due to the auto-splenectomy that often occurs.

G6PD deficiency: Oxidative stress like drugs, infx, & fava beans causes hemolysis due to ↓ Glutathione reduction.

Work up: blood smear, which will show Heinz bodies.

Tx: supportive due to self-limitation of the disease. If the cause of the attack was infx, treat the infx. Advise the pt to avoid the causative drug or fava beans. G6PD test in RBC can be falsely elevated in the acute hemolysis due to the high level of reticulocytes & young RBCs. Therefore, the best time for the test is after a few weeks of supportive Tx & when Sx of jaundice & anemia have resolved.

Autoimmune hemolysis: either warm antibodies (IgG) seen w/ extravascular hemolysis or cold antibodies (IgM) seen w/ intravascular hemolysis. You diagnose autoimmune hemolytic anemia w/ a direct antiglobulin test, better known as the Coombs test. You will do this when you have a pt w/ a known hemolytic anemia, & you need to know if it is immune-mediated. This test tells you if there are antibodies or complement bound to the RBCs, because Coombs' reagent is an antibody against human antibodies. Therefore, if a RBC is covered in IgG (warm), Coombs' reagent binds to these, clumps together & causes the blood to clot. An antibody against complement is also added, & will do the same thing if there is complement covering the RBCs (as in IgM, cold).

Warm autoimmune hemolytic anemia: the body begins to make IgG antibodies that stick to the pt's own RBCs. This labels the RBCs for destruction by macrophages in the spleen, which is called extravascular hemolysis. It is called warm because these antibodies work best at warm temperatures, i.e. 37°C (or 98. 6°F-the body temperature). The most common etiology behind this is idiopathic. However, there are times where the body is making antibodies against lymphomas, autoimmune diseases such as SLE, & meds (like PCN), & the antibodies also recognize the pt's RBCs. Pts will NOT only present w/ the normal signs & Sx of hemolytic anemia, but also w/ splenomegaly. Tx includes eradicating the cause (such as the PCN), steroids, or splenectomy (in refractory cases), as the spleen is the source of the hemolysis in these cases. **Cold autoimmune hemolytic anemia:** IgM antibodies cause intravascular hemolysis when the temperature drops below 37°C (by complement fixation). The etiologies include *mycoplasma pneumoniae*, infectious mononucleosis, along w/ idiopathic & lymphomas. Tx includes cold avoidance. Steroids usually are NOT effective. Rituximab is usually effective for both types but it is NOT the 1st option.

Microangiopathic hemolytic anemia: This is a small vessel disease where the RBCs are ripped apart by physical trauma. You should consider this when you have intravascular hemolysis & schistocytes (fragmented RBCs) on the blood smear (very important tool for diagnosing anemia in general). The trauma usually occurs from the RBCs getting ripped as they try to pass through a small vessel that has been crowded w/ a fibrin mesh. It can also occur when the RBCs are getting crushed from some sort of abnormal flow, such as in a mechanical heart valve, malignant HTN, or coarctation of the aorta. In the case of the fibrin-laden small vessels, there is usually a cause behind the ↑ activation of the Coagx pathway that leads to the hemolysis, such as DIC, preeclampsia/HELLP syndrome, HUS (hemolytic uremic syndrome), & TTP (thrombotic thrombocytopenic purpura).

Drug-induced hemolysis: consider when a new meds is administered, & then see signs & Sx of hemolytic anemia (jaundice, anemia, ↑ indirect bilirubin, ↑ LDH)

Work up for all hemolytic anemia: Order a CBC w/ reticulocyte count (RC), CMP (has total bili), hemolysis labs (direct bili/LDH/haptoglobin/urine hemosiderin/coombs antibodies), & peripheral smear. In hemolysis, labs will show r reticulocytes, ↑ LDH, ↑ indirect bilirubin (total bili – direct bili), & ↓ haptoglobin. A Coombs test (the direct & indirect) will be positive w/ antibody-mediated hemolysis. Urine hemosiderin is positive w/ intravascular hemolysis.

Special consideration:

- **The most common types are homozygous SS anemia (Hgb SS is the most severe).** There are other heterozygous conditions (Hgb SC or S-B thalassemia). SS trait (meaning they only have 1 abnormal allele in the recessive disease) is present in 8-10% of African Americans & is usually w/o Sx.
- ↑ **WBC (10-20k) & platelets (>450k)** are common due to overstimulation of bone marrow & auto-splenectomy.
- **Excessive IV fluid administration, along w/ pregnancy** can cause dilutional anemia (WBC & platelets will be down too). Excessive lab draws for blood work in long hospitalizations can cause anemia as well.
- **Pure RBC transfusion is usually needed if the Hgb<7** unless pt has Sx (like CP for coronary artery disease pts, etc) so you need to consider transfusion even if Hgb 7-10
- **Iron deficiency anemia w/o a known reason** (like heavy menstrual periods or multiple pregnancies for premenopausal pts) is an indication for colonoscopy to r/o a possible GI malignancy oozing blood especially for pts >50 years old.
- **Assess appropriate response post-transfusion.** 1 unit RBCs transfused is expected to ↑ the Hgb 1 g/dL.
- **Jehovah's witnesses:** do NOT usually accept any blood transfusion due to strict religious believes. NOT all Jehovah's Witnesses feel the

same way about transfusion; some may allow that. So talk w/ the pt (in privacy) & make sure you know the pt's wishes. Minimize blood withdrawal & use pediatrics tube as needed.

42. Night float

This is a quick snap shot of the most common calls you may encounter while you are covering in pt nights. More comprehensive details are discussed in other sections.

Chest pain: **always examine the pt**. Consider in your differential diagnosis problems, which could be catastrophic to miss such as MI, pulm embolism/DVT, & pneumothorax. Do the appropriate exam & consider EKG, troponin, CXR, ABG (if there is dyspnea or desaturation on pulse Ox), O_2 mask, & D-dimer (discouraged to use for in pt).

> **Attention**: Consider heparin drip, ASA, NTG, morphine prn if NOT contraindicated according to your initial evaluation if you suspect ACS. Consider heparin drip also even before CTA if you highly suspect pulm embolism (immobility, tachypnea, tachycardia, & desaturation) & the rest of exam did NOT indicate otherwise.

Abdominal pain: **always examine the pt**. R/o surgical abdomen & other associated sx, which may indicate causes other than simple indigestion (like N/V, fever, diarrhea, diaphoresis & ↓ appetite). Consider EKG if high suspicion for inferior MI. Abdominal X-ray can show SBO (air/fluid levels), ileus (severely sick/opioids), fecal impaction (solid fecal material on the left abdomen). Consider PPI, Pepto-Bismol, pain meds as indicated & treat the underlying problem.

Fever: Consider CBC w/ diff, blood Cx, Urinalysis (UA) & urine Cx, CXR, & starting/adding/switching Abx. Examine the pt & see what is indicated. Usually if the fever is the only sign w/o cough, sputum, HA, nuchal rigidity, AMS, urinary Sx, abdominal pain, consider doing them all. Fever w/ AMS may need lumbar puncture (LP)

& /or CT scan of head w/ contrast (r/o meningitis especially if focal neuro deficits are present).
If there is a known reason for fever like PNA or abscess & the pt is on the right abx, you can consider giving Tylenol (abx may need 1-2 days to fully work). That is unless the pt was afebrile for 24 hrs & then spiked a fever again; then you may need to send another set of cultures & possibly switch/add abx (may be resistant bug).

Insomnia: check sleep hygiene (avoid day napping, adequate daylight exposure, eating close to the sleeping time, caffeine intake, relaxing bedtime routine w/ less excessive night activities). Environmental changes like opening the curtains for light in the morning or sitting on bed or chair w/ physical therapy & early mobility in the morning may help. Use low dose benzos (like ambien or ativan) cautiously & temporarily especially in elderly (better to use mirtazapine or olanzapine/zolpidem) & it is better if you could avoid meds.

Critical electrolytes result:

- **Hypokalmia:** replaced by PO Kcl 10, 20, 40, 80 meq (tastes bad & could cause N/V & GI upset) or IV (called minibag) Kcl 10, 20 meq (dose 20 needs central line due to irritation, one bag usually takes 1-2 hrs). Usually each 10 meq PO or IV replaces 0. 1 of K in the blood. So if pt's K is 2. 8, give at least 70 to 100 meq (especially if you have hypokalemic-inducing factors like loop diuretics or vomiting). Check EKG (T wave flattening) & assess the route & urgency for K replacement. Keep it above 4 meq especially in CHF pts due to diuretic use.

- **Hyperkalemia:** give Kayexalate PO, which is a non-absorbable ion-exchange resin in GI system (it can be given by enema if NOT tolerating PO). Usually it takes hrs to work (can cause intestinal necrosis; avoid postoperatively & if constipation existed/ developed). You can give insulin & D5 fluids & Ca gluconate (stabilize the myocardium membrane & protect from arrhythmias) in case of EKG changes (T wave peaking). HD to ↓ K is always an option especially for pts already on HD. EKG changes → Ca gluconate + above options.

- **Hypocalcemia:** look at the albumin first & correct the Ca results (as the albumin carries the Ca & it can give pseudohypocalcemia in case of hypoalbuminemia). The correction factor is to add 0.8mg to the total Ca for each 1g drop in albumin. Normal low Ca is 8. 2 & normal low albumin is 3. 2, so if Ca is 7mg & albumin is 2g, no need to replace Ca. PO Ca is $CaCo_3$ & IV Ca is Ca gluconate (1-2 gr IV is the usual replacement dose). You can check ionized Ca for critical pts & no need for albumin correction in that case.
- **Hypophosphatemia:** PO form is Neutraphos & IV form is K-phos or Na-phos & dose is autocalculated.
- **Hypomagnesemia:** Mg oxide PO (comes as 400, 800mg) & Mg sulfate IV (dose is mostly autocalculated). Keep it above 2mg especially in CHF pts due to diuresis use. Milk of Magnesia (Mg hydroxide is a laxative)

Constipation: look for abdominal pain, abdominal distention, guarding (or any sign of surgical abdomen), N/V. Ask about PMH & meds which could cause constipation or ileus & electrolytes for hypercalcemia or hypokalemia which may cause constipation. If any of these alarming Sx are positive, proceed w/ treating underlying issue or call surgery if surgical abdomen presented (usually it is NOT surgical/ileus is NOT surgical). Digital rectal exam can be helpful to check for stool impaction (could be therapeutic as well). In general, if chronic, consider docusate, milk of magnesia, MiraLax (all PO). You can use water enema or Bisacodyl suppositories. If acute constipation, consider ruling out

SBO, volvulus, ileus, new opioid use w/o laxatives by ordering abdominal X-ray & if negative, proceed w/ as above.

A fib w/ RVR: **always examine the pt,** usually HR>110-120 & it needs an urgent action as the pt could develop tachycardia-related cardiomyopathy if left untreated even if asymptomatic. Check BP & ask about CP, feeling of palpitation, dizziness, blurry vision, & SOB. If any is present, consider urgent/emergent electric cardioversion. If not, try to slow the heart w/ : PO metoprolol, PO diltiazem, IV, metoprolol (10mg) bolus, IVdiltiazem bolus (20mg q15minute in general or 0. 25mg/kg for low body weight), & IV amiodarone. Consider anticoagx according to CHADS2 score but it is NOT as urgent as controlling the rate. Consider MICU transfer if RVR is refractory to PO meds & IV boluses for IV continuous drip meds like diltiazem or amiodarone.

Headache HA: Tylenol is great for HA. Ask for the chronicity of the HA, acute onset is more concerning than chronic. R/o by hx, "the worst HA in my life" (SAH), focal neurological deficits by appropriate neuro exam (r/o CVA), fall/trauma (r/o Intracranial IC bleeding) & nuchal rigidity/fever (meningitis). Ask what meds the pt takes usually for his/her HA. Stress HA is a common type & responds to simple Tylenol. Consider CT scan if indicated.

Itching: Broad DDx (uremia, cirrhosis, idiopathic, etc). R/o allergic reaction, review meds & stop the new ones, which may be the culprit. Assess for anaphylactic Sx like SOB/tongue edema & respond as appropriate (IV epinephrine, IV Solu-Medrol, IV Benadryl & consider intubation/ENT consult). Relieve w/ Benadryl or Atarax (PO or IV). Think about a more serious diagnosis when you see alarming signs like skin ulcers, rash, fever, boluses (dermatology consult for TSS or Steven Johnson Syndrome).

Nausea & vomiting: If these are new Sx, ask about other related Sx like abd. Pain, diarrhea, constipation, CP, fever or possible DKA picture & evaluate/treat as indicated. Symptomatic management w/ PO/IV Zofran, Phenergan & Reglan.

Fall: **always examine the pt,** ask about how it happened, where, witnesses, Coagx status, from how high, head trauma, LOC, N/V, focal neuro deficits, vision/pupils, & skeletal tenderness. If neuro exam is NOT changed from before, no LOC, no other signs of intracranial bleeding: neuro exam q1h for a few hrs afterwards by an MD or a nurse may be enough (although you can do CT scan w/o contrast if you have a high concern even w/ negative exam). Document your evaluation, order CT scan head, & bone x-rays, & prescribe pain meds as indicated.

Altered Mental Status (AMS): **always examine the pt,** broad DDx. In general, make sure vitals are stable, O_2 sat & CBG are okay, look for infx signs like UTI, PNA or bacteremia as indicated, check the admission diagnosis as it may be related to the AMS like fever in elderly. If your initial exam is normal, give PO/IV haldol, PO/IM Olanzapine (for elderly), PO/IV Ativan (avoid benzos for elderly). Consider wrist strains if they are at risk to harm themselves like pulling IV lines. Consider EtOH withdrawal & give PRN ativan (they may need high doses)

Hypo/hyperglycemia: Hypo is more serious than hyper due to neurological impairment, which can be caused by hypoglycemia especially for a long term. Check for sympathetic Sx like tachycardia, diaphoresis, AMS, & tremors for hypoglycemia. Give PO juice, cookies, 50cc D50 IV bolus (or called amp) or even IV D5 or D10 depending on responsiveness & Sx & ↓ insulin dose. Try NOT to hold long acting insulin (lantus or NPH) in case of corrected hypoglycemia episode. For hyperglycemia, calculate the correction factor (CF) & give fast acting insulin (regular or aspart), which is usually called supplemental or sliding scale.

Shortness of Breath/Hypoxia/Hypercapnia: always examine the pt. Broad DDx, usually comes together & the evaluation is usually similar. In general, think about pulm embolism ($\downarrow O_2$ $\downarrow CO_2$), pulm edema (excessive IV fluid/CHF), excessive respiratory secretions (deep suction resolves Sx quickly), worsening COPD/asthma/PNA (wheezing & consolidation), Pneumothorax (especially if they had recent lung procedure like thoracentesis/bronchoscopy/central line), recent blood transfusion in the last 24 hrs (Transfusion Related Acute Lung Injury (TRALI)). Consider O_2 masks, NIV (non-invasive ventilation, which is a tight mask to deliver more O_2), intubation, CXR, ABG, troponin, CBC, lactic acid, MICU consult, lasix, morphine as indicated (follow ACLS algorithm if pt is unstable).

Special consideration:
- **Call upper level in case of complicated picture** for second opinion.
- **Assess for the need for MICU transfer** in case of hemodynamic instability, hard to manage on the floor (due to need of intubation or IV drip for heart rate control in case of A fib w/ RVR for instance), need for q1hr CBG in case of refractory hypoglycemia, alcohol withdrawal Sx need a lot of Ativan (usually >10 mg in last 24h) or any other problem may need an ICU evaluation.
- **Giving too much O_2 in COPD pt causes respiratory depression (common mistake)** since respiratory drive is controlled by hypoxemia (normal person have the respiratory drive from hypercapnia which is NOT working for COPD pts due to chronic CO_2 retention). So a lot of O_2 is bad for COPD pts who retain CO_2 (O_2 sat between 88-92% is may be acceptable).

Chronic hypercapnia may NOT feel the sedation effect of CO_2 until $PaCO_2$ >90-100 while normally sedation is noted when $PaCO_2$ 60-70.

- **Mg, K, & Ca are connected & need to be corrected simultaneously:** Mg is needed in order for parathyroid gland to sense hypocalcemia & secrete PTH. The kidney tries to keep Mg in blood (in hypomagnesemia) & excrete K in urine in that process. That makes hypocalcemia & hypokalemia refractory to replacement if Mg is NOT corrected first.
- **Do EKG first** when you have K or Ca abnormality & correct faster in case of T wave changes.

43. Alarming findings

These following findings may indicate a serious diagnosis requiring fast action to prevent imminent morbidity & mortality or would indicate or require further management due to possible hidden serious disease.

- **GERD w/ dysphagia,** odynophagia, weight loss, anemia, GI bleed, long term GERD, & old age (>50) requires an upper endoscopy to r/o Barrett's esophagus & adenocarcinoma.
- **Neutropenia w/ fever** (>38.3 c) requires pan-cultures (to seek out the infx source), CXR (PNA), urine analysis (UTI), & empiric abx (Vanc, Zosyn, & possibly fluconazole).
- **Unexplained microcytic anemia** requires colonoscopy to r/o colon cancer.
- **Benign prostatic hypertrophy w/ back pain** requires back X-ray & PSA test due to suspicion of prostate cancer.
- **Known ulcerative colitis w/ abdominal pain & fever** high suspicion for toxic megacolon & requires an abdominal X-ray. You may also consider treating w/ ↑ dose IV steroids & consulting surgery.
- **Anorexia, cachexia, weight loss, & lymphadenopathy** are suspicious signs for cancer & age appropriate cancer screening should be done.
- **Change in stool caliber** may indicate distal colon cancer & should be alarming. Consider colonoscopy, especially if >50 years old or family hx of colon cancer (look for microcytic anemia for another clue).
- **Back pain w/** incontinence & saddle paresthesia indicates spinal cord compression. This requires a high dose IV steroid; radiotherapy & a surgery consult ASAP (make sure you get Biopsy mostly by IR to help in diagnoses if cancer is suspected).

- **HAs w/ temporal tenderness** may indicate Giant cell arteritis & it may requires high dose IV steroids. To prevent blindness, begin steroids before waiting for elevated ESR lab results.
- **CP w/ ST segment elevation** requires cards consult & cath lab (or thrombolytics depending on the facility) & giving urgent medicine in a short time frame (revascularization in <90 minutes). Urgent meds: ASA 325, plavix 600, Heparin drip, metoprolol (if SBP>100), NTG SQ, SL, IV (if NOT contraindicated), O_2 (if desating), morphine prn (if still in pain after NTG).
- **Asthma or COPD exacerbation pts who canNOT make a complete sentence** due to their SOB require immediate action. Administer O_2, jet nebs (Ventolin & ipratropium), & IV steroids. Consider a stat ICU evaluation while awaiting ABGs & CXR results if pt's Sx do NOT improve (for possible intubation).

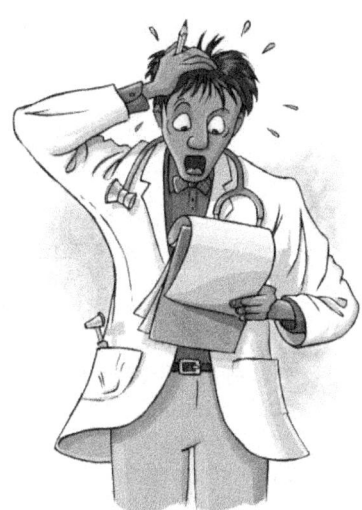

Some signs may be alarming for another serious condition; recognize those signs.

44. IV lines, IV fluids, Foley catheters & contrast material

IV lines: Most of the hospital pts need peripheral IV lines for IV meds, blood draws, fluids, blood, or resuscitation in case of dehydration or bleeding (sometimes you need 2 large bore peripheral IV lines for faster fluid resuscitation).

Central lines (intra-jugular & peripherally inserted central cath PICC) are indicated for the following: long-term hospitalization (blood withdrAwal), delivery of certain meds maybe NOT appropriate peripherally (e.g. 20 meq K or >D5% fluid), critical pts w/ HoTN & needing vasopressors, small peripheral veins or "hard stick", & long term IV therapy (e.g., infective endocarditis requiring IV abx for 6 weeks).

> **Attention:** Be cautious w/ HD pts as they may need any possible dialysis port access & any central IV access should be done per nephrology recommendations (except in emergencies).

Fluids: Most commonly used are Normal Saline (NS), Dextrose 5% water (D5W), D5 NS, D5 1/2NS.

Fluid replacement: In cases of fluid deficits, which can manifest w/ HoTN or tachycardia due to bleeding (internal or external), dehydration (sweating, excessive diuresis, diarrhea, etc), & septic shock (no frank fluid deficits & it is more of ↓ vessels resistance).

The rate of correction of volume depletion depends upon severity. For pts w/ severe volume depletion or hypovolemic shock, we recommend administration of 1 to 2 liters of isotonic saline as rapidly as possible (~999cc/hr) in an attempt to restore tissue perfusion. Fluid repletion is continued at a rapid rate until the clinical signs of hypovolemia improve (eg, ↓ blood pressure, tachycardia, ↓ urine output, impaired mental status or up trending of lactic acid).

For pts w/ CHF you can do 250cc or 500cc boluses & evaluate for pulm edema in between by assessing SOB & breath sounds (intubate as needed).

Maintenance fluid: In cases of NPO status, where pt canNOT tolerate PO intake for any reason (eg, pancreatitis, gastroenteritis). Usually it is 75-100ml/h & total of 2 L/day (which is going to be equal to the insensible water loss in sweat, metabolism, & stool, as well as minimal urinary output). This rate, however, is NOT sufficient for replacing any fluid deficits/hypovolemia/dehydration & it is usually after to replace the deficits aggressively as above.

Special consideration:

- **Free water flushes (through NG tube)** can be considered for Tx of hypernatremia. Giving fluids through the GI system is preferred over IV unless it is urgent.
- **Reassess the need for IV fluids on a daily bases** to prevent iatrogenic pulm edema especially for pts w/ CHF (systolic or diastolic/preserved EF). Euvolemic pts who are tolerating PO intake do NOT need IV fluids.
- **Be aware of dilutional anemia** (↓ in RBC, WBC & platelets).
- **HoTN refractory** to the initial 2-3 L fluids resuscitation may indicate the need for MICU transfer & BP support meds (epinephrine/phenylephrine/vasopressin/norepinephrine). In general, the need for 3 or more BP support meds indicates very poor prognosis. HoTN refractory to fluid resuscitation differentiates sepsis (HoTN respond to IV fluid & no need for vasopressors) from septic shock (persistent HoTN despite IV fluid & need Vasopressors).

- **Some conditions require a lot of fluid resuscitation** (>4-6L of NS in the first 6 hrs), such as DKA, HHNS, pancreatitis, severe dehydration, & septic shock.

Foley catheter: ↑ the risk of UTI & needs daily assessments in deciding to whether to continue or to discontinue. It is indicated for urinary retention (like BPH) & strict ins/outs monitoring, especially when assessing a CHF pt's response to diuresis or assessing a shock pt's response to fluid resuscitation (consider a condom cath for cooperative men w/ no obstruction/still ↑ UTI risk to 2folds).
Other pts requiring intake/output monitoring include: critically ill pts, perioperative pts, & end-of-life pts needing palliative care.
Bladder scans (better) or in/out Foley cath can differentiate between urinary retention & anuria (no urine in the bladder like in AKI). Consider a Foley cath in place if the scan shows >350-400cc post voidal residual urine (means urinary retention).
Urine culture from indwelling foley cath may NOT be accurate due to colonization (which does NOT indicate abx use).

Contrast material (IV): CT (Iodine based) or MRI (Gadolinium) w/ IV contrast is useful when you are looking for infx or cancer. Contrast induced nephropathy can occur w/ already damaged kidney (CKD at any stage). If IV contrast is essential in a pt w/ mildly elevated Cr, you can use Acetylcysteine (both prior & post-study) & aggressive IV hydration (NS 200-250 cc/hr) prior to contrast administration.

Special consideration:
- **Gadolinium should be avoided in ESRD** even if on HD due to the risk of nephrogenic systemic fibrosis (NSF), thickening of the skin & other organs.
- **Barium contrast (NOT water soluble)** administered PO or rectally along w/ X-ray or CT can evaluate for

GI pathology. Gastrografin (water soluble) should be used as contrast material if you suspect perforated esophagus.

- **Cardiac catheterization w/ IV contrast** is a common procedure. Kidney function should be monitored before & after the procedure (usually in the next 24 hrs) for AKI ($\uparrow$ in Cr >30% of the baseline).
- **Try to avoid using two IV contrast studies** w/ in 24 hours period, like left heart cath & CTA (especially in case of kidney disease). Consider MRI as a second study if CT w/ contrast was done earlier at the same day (if possible).

45. Medicine facts (side effects, onset of side effects, & off-label therapeutic uses)

Common facts for common meds commonly used:

- **QT interval prolongation:** can be caused by a lot of meds like quinolones, antiarrhythmic meds (amiodarone/tykosin/procainamide), psychiatry meds (fluoxetine/quetiapine/haldol), pain meds (methadone), & a lot of others. This can evolve to torsades de pointes (TdP), which is a unique V tachycardia. Monitor QTc before & on a regular basis after starting & consider stopping the meds if QTc >500-550. Check K & Mg & replete as needed. Treat TdP w/ ↑ dose IV Mg along w/ ACLS.
- **Statins:** ↑ Creatine kinase (from muscles) & AST/ALT. Statins can help maintaining sinus rhythm after a fib cardioversion (ACE inhibitors can help as well maintaining sinus rhythm), but it is still NOT used for that purpose alone.
- **Pregnancy & antiemetics:** non-pharmacological methods are preferred like eating small meals, avoiding strong odors, getting enough sleep, & avoiding fatigue. Evidence is insufficient regarding the safety of most of the meds. Many class C antiemetic meds are prescribed during pregnancy when benefits> risks. **Meds:** multivitamins, Zofran, Phenergan, Reglan, & Meclizine.
- **Cirrhosis & Tylenol:** up to 2 g/day is safe (up to 4g/day in healthy person). Toxicity is when levels are up to 10-15 g/day. Acetylcysteine is the antidote.
- **Cirrhosis & increased Ammonia:** Use Lactulose (laxatives, monitor) & Rifaximine (abx). NO need to monitor Ammonia levels &

follow up clinical response (up titrate lactulose dose to target 3-4 bowel movements)

- **Pulmonary HTN & Remodulin (**peripheral prostacyclin vasodilator) infusion pump: do NOT hold because rebound pulm HTN may occur & could be catastrophic.
- **Metoprolol & Coreg for A fibTx:** both can rate control the heart. Coreg has alpha-1 blocking activity & can cause HoTN (metoprolol causes less HoTN). So choose coreg if you want to control HTN along w/ slowing the rate.

> **Attention**: max β blocker and ACEi doses for CHF pts before adding another CHF meds to get the mortality benefits (like 25bid for coreg and 40 for lisinopril).

- **Blood levels:** of some meds should be monitored to assure therapeutic levels & avoid toxicity. Check levels after starting new meds → change doses & /or start another med incase of drug-drug interaction. Examples: Vanc, Dilantin, Valproic acid, phenobarbital, tacrolimus, digoxin, lithium (some meds can cause the adverse effect even on therapeutic levels like brady or tachy arrhythmias w/ digoxin & lithium). Make sure you correct the phenytoin level for albumin in case of hypoalbuminemia (false low levels if albumin is low).
- **Nitroglycerin facts: 1.** NTG w/ Viagra can cause refractory HoTN. **2.** Do NOT give NTG if SBP is <90. **3.** NTG is used to relieve ischemic pain (up to 3 doses, 0. 4mg q5min), so no need for NTG if there is no pain. **4.** NTG is contraindicated for inferior MI since those pts are volume-dependent (actually sometime they require IV fluids to maintain BP). NTG will ↓ the preload which they will NOT tolerate (treat HoTN w/ IV fluids)

- **Changes in thyroxine** replacement therapy for hypothyroidism require 4-6 weeks to affect the TSH levels. Small changes in TSH in the in-pt setting do NOT require synthroid dose adjustments. **In general:** do NOT adjust thyroxine dose for pts in the hospital as TSH changes is maybe just from sick thyroid syndrome & may be misleading (repeat TSH in few weeks if abnormal).
- **Warfarin** is a common anticoagx medicine & requires continuous INR monitoring in warfarin clinic or, for selective pts, at home.
- **Morphines & narcotics (as well as benzodiazepines/sedatives in general)** can cause respiratory suppression for pts who already have underlying disorders like COPD & pulm fibrosis. Use w/ caution (avoid for pts w/ baseline hypoactive delirium to avoid intubation due to inability to protect airways).
- **PPI** (or H2 blocker) for GI & **heparin sq** for DVT prophylaxis are commonly used in the hospital pts. They are specifically important for ICU pts due to ↓ mobility & NPO status.

> **Attention**: to NOT start heparin on bleeding pt (like GI bleeding), while no real contraindication for PPI. May be PPI is NOT needed for pts admitted for observation for any reason if they are eating normally. PPI ↑ PNA risk.

- **Clonidine** is α1 agonist & is used for HTN. In the ICU, it can be used as a sedative agent (like Precedex but NOT commonly used for that purpose)
- **Clindamycin** can is strongly associated with C diff diarrhea but it can be a direct effect from the medicine itself, stop the medicine & test for C diff if diarrhea did NOT improve. It covers CA-

MRSA & it has anti-toxin quality (from toxin producing organism like strep) make it preferred for mild-moderate out or even in pt cellulitis Tx (small % of strep developed resistance to clindamycin; reassess & switch abx prn)

- **Bactrim** has K sparing ability in the kidney like sprinolactone & therefore can cause hyperkalemia.

> **Attention**: to hyperkalemia when Bactrim is used with other meds like ACEi & sprinolactone.

- **SSRI can cause SIADH** (hyponatremia w/o edema usually).
- **Loop diuretics & Na/ urine osmolarity:** although loop diuretics affect Na reabsorption (as thiazides); hyponatremia is less comparing to thiazides due to the higher urine osmolarity & Na concentration with thiazides (different mechanism of action). Maybe it is safe to assume that urine is hypertonic with thiazides & hypo or isotonic with loops. Ethacrynic acid is a loop diuretic but does NOT contain sulfa.
- **"Steroid taper":** usually prescribed for short period of time (like for COPD or Asthma) after giving moderate-high doses of steroids for >7-10 days (moderate-high prednisone dose is ≥20mg/day) to prevent pituitary-adrenal axis suppression. No need for that taper if the steroid dose is small (like 5 mg prednisone daily) or the high dose is <7days. No specific guidelines for steroid taper & it is mostly provider dependent.

Example: Prednisone 60mg for 3 days, 40mg for 3 days, 20mg for 3days, 10mg for 3 days & 5mg for 3 days & then stop. "Steroid taper" can be indicated also for different reason as a part of the therapy like to prevent frequent COPD exacerbations.

- **Common steroids comparison (w/doses)**

Hydrocortisone	Prednisone	Dexamethasone
20mg equal to	5mg equal to	1mg
High mineral & low anti-inflammatory activity (good for shock).	Medium mineral & medium anti-inflammatory activity	Low mineral & high anti-inflammatory activity (good for Cancer).

- **Pyridium:** is urinary analgesic for UTI, changes urine color normally to red/orange (inform the pt), use for short period (<2-3 days), avoid in case of AKI/CKD.

- **Antipsychotics:** used for positive Sx like delirium, psychosis (schizophrenia or mania) or negative Sx like flat affect or social withdrawal. 1st Gen. like Haldol has antidopamine effect & it is safer for elderly (w/ dementia) & cardiac pts while 2nd Gen. are antidopamine & serotonin (& anticholinergic as a side-effect) like Olanzapine ($\uparrow$ appetite & $\uparrow$ blood sugar) /Seroquel ($\uparrow$ appetite & help sleeping)/Abilify ($\downarrow$ appetite & least anticholinergic)/Clozapine (cause agranulocytosis & used after 2 other antipsychotic fail). Both have the same antipsychotic effect but 2nd gen. help in negative Sx (unlike 1st Gen.). Look for the long acting forms (injections) when adherence is a problem.

- **Estrogen & Desmopressin (DDAVP):** help in improving coagulation in case of bleeding disorders like in liver disease. DDAVP $\uparrow$ Von

235

willebrand factor release from endothelial cells. Use **Fibrin spray (Tisseel)** for superficial bleeding due to hemostatic effect.

- **Atropine:** can be indicated in symptomatic bradycardias like in heart blocks & it works by ↓ the parasympathic pathway → ↑ sympathic pathway. Due to the special heart innervation system (atriums→ parasympathic & sympathic but ventricles→just sympathic), atropine (works on parasympathic) may NOT work if the AV node is NOT conducting (consider pacemaker).
- **Always check** if any medicine you will prescribe needs to be **renally dosed** in case of AKI/CKD/ESRD. Do the same with Cirrhosis pts.
- **Allergic cross-reactivity:** angioedema from ACEi has ≈ 10% risk of allergy w/ ARBs & also anaphylactic from penicillin has ≈ 10% risk of allergy w/ cephalosporin & ≈ 1% w/ Aztreonam.

46. Medical vs. Surgical Management

This is a very important topic, & most likely this will be life-saving if the pt is appropriately triaged to the correct service. Most of these pts will be evaluated in the Emergency room, & sometimes the pt can develop complications on the floor, especially in our oncology population. Therefore, this topic will address key diseases where early diagnosis for medical or surgical management is critical. Don't forget just because the abdominal pain is NOT pronounced, does NOT mean it is NOT life threatening. Always think about the surgical options for treating any medical case & know when they can help.

Pancreatitis: Diagnosed w/ elevated lipase (more specific) & amylase (more sensitive). Always perform the Modified Ranson's criteria on admission & at 48 hrs (**available online**) to estimate mortality. Most common causes are EtOH & gallstones (worse), as well as, elevated triglyceride or Ca. If concerned for diagnosis is unclear or you want to r/o necrotizing pancreatitis→ obtain CT scan abdomen, which is NOT necessary for diagnoses. Surgical management along w/ GI consultation is always merited in cases of worsening necrotizing pancreatitis or unresolved pseudocysts (usually after wall cysts maturation, if possible).

> **Attention:** Amylase and lipase are useful in only making pancreatitis diagnosis (>3 times elvation of normal limits). However it does not indicate the severity of the pancreatitis and should NOT be followed for monitoring the pt improvement or worsening

Medical management of acute or acute on chronic pancreatitis is appropriate w/ mild disease, which subsides in a few days. The pancreas is given rest, w/ I. V. Fluids. Ringer's Lactate is now the preferred fluid of choice in all pancreatitis pts. Morphine or meperidine should be given for pain control. Avoid TPN at all cases, even in severe pancreatitis. Instead, a post pyloric feeding tube (NJ tube) may be placed. Continue the clear liquid diet until diet can be advanced to regular diet (advance diet as soon as tolerated) when abdominal pain improves. If pancreatitis is caused due to biliary obstructions then, laparoscopic cholecystectomy might be performed during the in pt hospital stay.

Diverticulitis: is inflammation or infx of the diverticular pouches w/ fecal impaction that can lead to erosion & bowel perforation.

Management:

- Do **CT scan** to identify pts who are likely to respond to conservative medical therapy or will need surgery evaluation.
  Conservative Tx (Bowel rest w/ NPO or/& NJ tube & abx) in pts w/ uncomplicated diverticulitis → success rate is 70 – 100%.
- Decide **Out pt vs. In pt**: Severity of presentation, the ability to tolerate PO intake, the presence of comorbid diseases, & the available support system need to be taken into account. Hospitalization is required for immunosuppressed, the elderly, those w/ significant comorbidities, & those w/ ↑ fever or significant leukocytosis.
- **Abx:**
  In pt ABX: Average 10 – 14 days depending on resolution of Sx. Gram-negative rods & anaerobes (particularly *E. coli* & *Bacteroides fragilis*) are the usual causes of diverticulitis: Fluoroquinolones w/ metronidazole, Amoxicillin-clavulanate, or TMP-SMX w/ metronidazole are the options.

Out pt: 10 – 14 day of Ciprofloxacin & metronidazole. Ciprofloxacin is the best option because it has better coverage of gram-negative pathogens. **Another option** is Amoxicillin-clavulanate. If NOT tolerable to metronidazole use Clindamycin/moxifloxacin.

- 6 weeks after recovery pts should undergo a colonoscopy to exclude other diagnosis. Considerations such as colonic neoplasia & to evaluate the extent of the diverticulosis.
- **Surgery Indications:**
  Absolute indication: Complications of diverticulitis (peritonitis, abscess, fistula, obstruction), clinical deterioration or failure to improve w/ medical therapy, recurrent episodes, intractable Sx (sepsis), or inability to exclude carcinoma. Recurrence diverticulitis rate is 35%
- **Surgical goals:** remove the septic focus by resection of the colon, treat obstruction or fistula, & restore bowel continuity (while minimizing morbidity & mortality).
- **Laparoscopic vs. open resection:**
  Laparoscopic surgeries are associated w/ a shorter recovery time. Fast-track recovery protocols improve perioperative outcomes in pts for whom elective laparoscopic surgery is performed. Shorter time to consuming a soft diet (2. 3 vs. 3. 6 days), 1st bowel movement (2. 6 vs. 3. 5 days), median length of hospital stay (3 vs. 5 days), & lower morbidity (15 vs. 26%) compared w/ pts managed w/ traditional postoperative care.

Aortic Aneurysm: is an enlargement of the aorta to greater than 1. 5 times normal size. While the cause of an aneurysm may be multifactorial, the end result is an underlying weakness in the wall of the aorta at that location. These pts are very tricky in that if they are stable then they do NOT meet surgery indication, but when they are too sick, they are unstable for surgery. It can be very challenging to treat these pts.

Asymptomatic pts w/ AAA diameter < 5. 5 cm: unlikely to rupture. Situations for which elective repair of AAA <5. 5 cm is considered:

- **Rapidly expanding**: Infrarenal AAA rapidly expanding in well-documented series of imaging. >0. 5 cm in six months or >1 cm per year. Rapid expansion may represent instability of the aortic wall, & some studies suggest that rapidly expanding AAAs have a higher risk of rupture.
- **Associated Arterial disease present:** coexisting iliac, femoral, or popliteal artery aneurysms, or Symptomatic peripheral artery disease.
- **Women** have higher risk of rupture than men. Elective repair of asymptomatic AAA >5 cm in females may be appropriate. However, the risk of death from elective repair is also ↑ in women. A lower threshold for repair is best reserved for women who have ↓ risk for perioperative morbidity & mortality.

Symptomatic AAA (abdominal/back/flank pain or limb ischemia): These Sx can be attributed to the aneurysm. Even w/ absence of overt rupture, the presence of Sx↑ the risk for AAA rupture. Only 50 % of people w/ ruptured AAA will reach the hospital & of these people 30 – 50% will die in spite of significant advances in intensive care unit management & surgical techniques.

Initial management of pts w/ Symptomatic (non-ruptured) & ruptured AAA: Place large bore peripheral intravenous lines for meds & fluid administration, manage their pain, & prepare them for surgery. For pts w/ ruptured AAA maintain the systolic blood pressure between 80 & 100 mmHg (permissive HoTN) rather than at higher levels prior to repair. Emergent surgery is indicated.

Cholelithiasis: (gallstone) is a concentration of crystalline product formed in the gallbladder by bile components. These calculi may pass distally into other parts of the biliary tract & cause obstruction, which leads to cholecystitis. These pts usually present w/ complaints of biliary colic & postprandial (particularly w/ fatty foods) right upper quadrant pain lasting a few hrs.

Medical Tx: mostly out pt, but can prescribe ursodeoxycholic acid (Ursodiol) therapy 300 mg BID for long-term management & pain control w/ NSAIDs. If the pt is experiencing recurrent cholelithiasis then elective cholecystectomy can be performed to prevent future attacks of biliary colic.

Acute cholecystitis: occurs most commonly due to obstruction. Pts may present acutely w/ RUQ pain, fever, leukocytosis, ↑ levels of ALK-P & GGT. Right upper quadrant ultrasound showing a thickened gallbladder wall & /or stones is diagnostic. Empiric abx (vanc/zosyn) should be started promptly on admission & given prior to surgery. Surgery is usually recommended w/ in the first 3 days of admission. In ↑ risk pts, or the ones who are too sick or unstable to undergo surgery, a percutaneous drainage device should be placed by Interventional Radiology along w/ abxTx.

Attention: to meds side effect in hyponatremia DDx.

Acute Cholangitis: is a biliary tract infx, usually caused by an infx building behind a stone obstruction. The pt presents w/ a triad of Sx: Fever + Jaundice + RUQ pain = Charcot's triad. If you add AMS + HoTN + Charcot's Triad = Reynolds's Pentad. Pt should have GI medicine along w/ surgery consult, & will most likely need ERCP & removal of the stone.

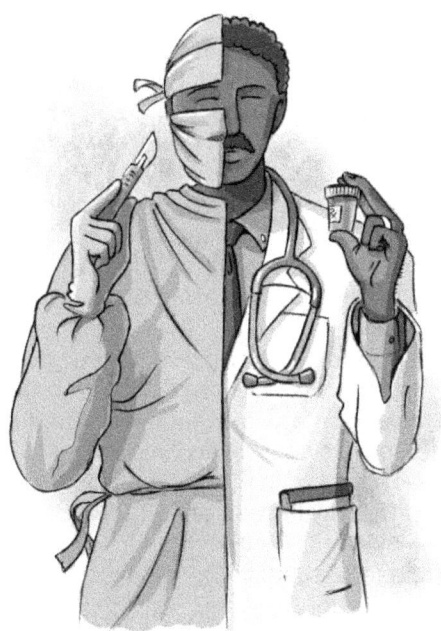

Surgery & medicine are complementary & needed for better pt's outcome.

Special consideration:

- **Hold strong pain meds to assess abdominal pain** progression so you do NOT miss catastrophic surgical event (in equivocal cases)
- **Septic knee effusion (septic joint) needs immediate arthrocentesis** to prevent long-term joint damage & help w/ diagnoses. Do NOT forget NPO if you suspect surgery or you have a pt w/ N/V & suspect bowl obstruction (consider NG tube).
- **Bowel ischemia** needs high suspicion & may need an emergent surgery consult to evaluate for bowel resection if it's NOT viable to prevent sepsis, f/u w/ lactic acid.

- **Trending Lactic acid** is helpful in case of any suspected ischemia (indicator of anaerobic metabolism). Reassuring if it is trending down
- **Empyema (pus in pleura, seen on chest ct scan) or abscess (in general)** needs drainage along w/ medical management. Pancreatitis & pancreatic cysts afterwards are commonly medically managed even if the necrotic tissue is up to 30% & surgery indication is very limited (in case of infected necrosis from CT scan guided FNA sample).
- **Other cases you can ask for surgical help when indicated:** Chronic osteomyelitis (ask vascular surgery to evaluate for amputation when perfusion is poor & refractory to abx), urinary obstruction (urology evaluation for nephrostomy in case of AKI), Pericardial effusion (for CT surgery evaluation in case of tamponade suspicion), spinal cord compression (Neurosurgery)
- **Pt's wishes are important to know** in case they do NOT want surgery so you can start/continue medical management ASAP
- **Assess the ability of lying flat:** for any surgical procedure as the anesthesia & surgery team will need to know that (CHF & COPD pts may NOT be able to lay flat &, therefore, will need different approaches)
- **Always get INR/PT/PTT/platelets count before any invasive procedure** or surgery to assess bleeding risk. Make sure pt is NPO at least 6-8 hrs before. ASA usually is fine to resume but in neurosurgery procedures. Plavix needs to be held for at least 5 days (to wash off).
- **Consider procedures:**
  HD for temporary use when necessary (AKI w/ refractory elevated K, refractory volume overload, ingestion of toxic material like ethylene glycol & so forth)

Bone marrow biopsy by HEM/ONC service to evaluate unexplained bloodline abnormalities or haematological malignancies

PICC line if you suspect long term IV route use (like endocarditis)

Consider interventional radiology consult in case of ↑ risk procedures like paracentesis, thoracentesis, LP, etc.

- **Preoperation cardiac risk stratification for non-cardiac surgery**: is commonly requested from either cardiology or internal medicine. The history, physical examination (especially cardiac), & EKG (looking for ischemic changes, arrhythmias, qwaves, or just to have a baseline) identify patient-specific risk factors. This information, combined with the surgery risk itself (high risk surgery: intrathoracic, cardiac, prolonged>4hrs, emergent & vascular surgeries. Low risk: Laparoscopic, endoscopic & eye procedures), is used to estimate perioperative risk of adverse cardiac events.

  There are various factors to be considered when assessing the cardiac risks of anesthesia & surgery. These are generally divided into patient-related & surgery-specific risks.

  In general: symptoms such as angina, dyspnea, syncope, & palpitations as well as a hx of heart disease including ischemic, valvular, arrhythmias or myopathic disease, & a hx of HTN, DM, CKD, & CVA or peripheral artery disease will ↑ the risk for major cardiac event during the surgery (MI or cardiac arrest).

  Cardiac functional status should be determined as well (how much METs pt can do as a baseline; **available online**). Usually walk up a flight of steps or a hill or walk on level ground at 3 to 4 mph (4 METs) is an acceptable/reassuring factor to go for an elective surgery (assuming no significant risk factors are present). Inability to climb two flights of stairs or walk four blocks ↑ risk of postoperative complications.

- There are **5 common scenarios for risk stratification** summarize most of the pts:

  1. Emergent non-cardiac surgery → go to OR (no need for cardiac testing); high risk

  2. Active cardiac Sx like SOB, arrhythmias, CP, CHF exacerbation, etc → No OR (treat the cardiac event appropriately); high risk

  3. Low risk surgery (regardless of other risk factors) → go to OR (no further testing); low risk

  4. Baseline METs ≥4 w/o active cardiac Sx (like ACS, CHF exacerbation, unstable arrhythmias, etc) → go to OR (no need for cardiac testing); pt's risk depends on the surgery risk itself (low, moderate, or high)

  5. METs ≤4 or unknown (orthopedic problem like amputation) → two scenarios:

  ≥3 risk factors (hx of CAD, valvular disease, arrhythmias, CHF, HTN, DM, CKD, & CVA or peripheral artery disease) or high risk surgery → No OR (get appropriate cardiac stress test or LHC to check for CAD & stent/CABG as indicated); high risk

  ≤2 risk factors → mostly go to OR (no further testing); low, moderate, or high risk depends on the surgery itself.

- **Giving β blocker anyway** for all pts going to surgery due to "cardiac protection" without pre existing indication (like known CAD, HTN, or CHF) is NOT indicated & did NOT show benefits (do NOT stop β blocker before surgery if pt was on it for any reason). Hold possible nephrotoxic meds like lisinopril or diuretics due to bleeding risk & HoTN

47. Home vs. floor vs. MICU triage

Triage: in the simplest terms means the process of determining the priority of pts' Tx based on the severity of their condition. This section is mainly focused to help interns triage on crossover, night float, & in the ICU. The 1st level of triaging is done by the emergency physicians, so we have to become familiar w/ their classification. Therefore, when they call for an admission we know the level of acuity based on the **Emergency Severity Index (ESI)** from **1** which indicate **severe** case (may need intensive care) to **5** which indicate **mild** case (may be managed in an out pt setting)

Example of ESI level 1: cardiac arrest, respiratory arrest, severe respiratory arrest, overdose w/ respiratory depression, hypoperfusion, anaphylactic shock, Symptomatic bradycardia, CP w/ hemodynamic instability.
Based on the ESI level 1 you know the pt will need a higher acuity of care, so these pts will go to the MICU, CCU, NICU, or a step down unit, if your hospital has one.
After the pt is triaged by the nursing staff, the pt is seen by the ER physician or resident, then medicine is called for evaluation of the pt either for admission, ICU placement, cardiology service, observation, or home.

> **Attention**: Always evaluate at the bedside in the ED & do NOT dismiss pts on the phone.

Based on lab values because labs might look ok, but the pt is not. See the pt, get a good H & P & use your clinical judgment. The emergency physicians are really busy, & they will NOT have the same time to get all the information.

If you feel the pt needs to be discharged, discuss w/ an upper level, fellow, or attending, then speak w/ the ER physician.

If the pt needs to go the ICU or cardiology service, justify your reasons & see if the ER physician will call Cardiology or MICU for evaluation before you admit. The ER physician's job is to provide acute care & send the pt to the proper service. Sometimes they need to get pts admitted fast to prevent ER boarding (overcrowding).

Special consideration:

- **Pneumonia:** good standard guide for admission is **CURB-65:** Confusion, Urea (BUN >20), Respiratory Rate >30, Blood pressure >90/60, Age >65. Score of 0-1: out pt, Score of 2: in pt wards, Score of 3 or greater: assess for ICU.
- **Diabetic ketoacidosis DKA: (**w/ elevated anion gap) needs ICU management (IV fluid, insulin, electrolytes control, etc) until the gap is closed & pt is switched from insulin drip to SQ when PO intake is tolerated.
- **Low systolic BP <90 w/ Sx (**make sure it is NOT chronic asymptomatic like in some dialysis pts) who are NOT responding to initial fluid challenge (like 1-2 Liter of NS), consider ICU evaluation for pressers use & close monitoring. Always know the vitals as most of the time your decision will be affected by them. Whoever you will discuss the pt w/ will want to know the vitals so he/she can forward their thinking.
- **Some interventions needs to be done in the ICU like:** IV β blocker or Ca blockers like metoprolol & diltiazem (for a fib & SVT), intubation & non-invasive ventilation, BP support infusion, arterial line placement for close BP monitoring, etc. Status post code-blue is a common ICU admission.

48. Outpatient Medicine

Important part of residency & it can be a future career. The following are some common pathology you may encounter in the clinic (Many others are included elsewhere in detail throughout the book).

Lipids: New guidelines for Tx are NOT totally depending on the actual lipid blood levels
- Start **high potency** statins on
  1. Individuals w/ clinical atherosclerotic cardiovascular disease (like CAD or CVA)
  2. Individuals w/ LDL-cholesterol levels ≥190.

- Start **moderate potency** statins on:
  1. Individuals w/ diabetes aged 40 to 75 years old w/ LDL-cholesterol levels between 70 & 189 mg/dL & w/o evidence of atherosclerotic cardiovascular disease.
  2. Individuals w/o evidence of cardiovascular disease or diabetes but who have LDL-cholesterol levels between 70 & 189 mg/dL & a 10-year risk of atherosclerotic cardiovascular disease (ASCVD calculator is available online)≥ 7. 5% (you can use high potency as well instead of moderate).

Statins:
High potency: Atorvastatin 40-80mg & Rosuvastatins 20-40mg (the goal is to achieve at least a 50% reduction in LDL).
Moderate potency: The rest of statins (like Simvastatins) including the high potency at lower doses (lowers LDL cholesterol 30% to 49%). Follow-up the lipid panel in 8-12 weeks after starting therapy & yearly afterwards. Get LFT as a baseline before therapy & another one in 3 months (acceptable to have elevated AST/ALT up to 3 times of normal limits). There is no need to repeat LFT unless clinically indicated (RUQ pain, ictrus, itching, etc).

Ostoartheritis (OA): Common, usually in the knees & cervical vertebrae. X-ray is a good initial test & usually the severity of the arthritis does NOT necessarily correlate w/ the severity of the Sx (mild arthritis could cause severe Sx & vice versa). Start Tylenol & NSAIDs if NOT contraindicated (CHF, GI bleeding, CKD, bleeding tendency, etc) & reevaluate. Consider further testing like MRI/CT scan if you expect a surgical intervention & refer to orthopedics. Usually stiffness from OA lasts<30minuts (Rheumatoid arthritis RA lasts>30m & has +RF, +CCP)

Lower back pain (LBP): #1 disability etiology in US for pts <40 yo. Acute <6 weeks while chronic >3 months. R/o serious diagnosis (need urgent referral to neurosurgery) like **Cauda Equina Syndrome** (ask about incontinence & saddle paresthesia & motor or sensory impairment) & **spinal stenosis** (pain on walking which relieved by rest →pseudoclaudication).
Hx & physical exam is essential to r/o **radical neuropathies** (pain radiating down the leg in a dermatome way, sensory & strength exam, including walking on toes & heals is warranted to localize the nerve involvement, L5/S1). **Muscle spasm** pain is very common (trauma or heavy lifting/exercising) which is usually very severe, sudden & disabling.
Tests: Imaging studies (CT or MRI are better than plan X-rays) in the first 4-6 weeks are not necessary unless **alarming Sx** present like hx of cancer (mets), illicit injection drugs (osteomyelitis or abscess), major neurologic deficits (disk problem), rest pain, systemic Sx like fever, & prolonged steroids use. Note that disk protrusion/heraniation ≠ back pain as bulging discs are seen in more than 50 percent of asymptomatic patients; asymptomatic herniated discs are seen as well, though less frequently.

Tx: pain meds as indicated in the pain meds ladder: Tylenol, NSAIDs, lortab, oxycodone, PO or IV morphine or dilaudid (for 1 month/no need for bed-rest/encourage exercise as tolerated). Know what meds that pt is taking at home & resume them as indicated (for hospital pts). **Consider high dose steroid** (Solu-Medrol IV) for spinal compression Sx & stat neurosurgery consult (or refer to them the chronic debilitating cases if the pt is willing surgery). **Conisder chiropractor & physical therapy** (for another 1 month if pain persist >1 month on pain meds). Refer to neurosurgery or neurology after 2 months of conservative Tx with pain meds & physical therapy. **Consider Psychological distress or secondary gains** for chronic LBP w/ "inappropriate pain" signs. Neck pain is very similar to LBP in management.

Infection:

- **URI:** presents w/ cough (may be w/ green/yellow sputum which does NOT necessarily means bacterial infx but could be viral), fever, & dyspnea. Viral mostly associated w/ runny nose, sneezing, conjunctivitis, sick contact & pt does NOT look very sick (viral is self-limited & treat supportively w/ 1st G antihistamine, cough meds, etc). If bacterial: Azithromycin (z pack) is a good option.
- **Pharyngitis/tonsillitis/sinusitis**: viral or bacterial. **CENTOR criteria**: can guide to start abx (mainly used for pharyngitis); as it is hard to differentiate between viral vs bacterial infx by just physical exam or radiology.

  Ask about 4 things:
  Fever>38c, cervical adenopathy, tonsillar exudates, & the absent of cough or rhinitis (calculator **available online**).

  If **0-1** present→ **no abx**
  2-3 → **rapid strep** swab test & if positive→ start abx (z pack or Augmentin),
  4→ **start abx** w/o further testing.

Palpate for sinus tenderness & do trans-illumination test of maxillary sinus (properly trans-illuminated in case of air→ normal; trans illumination is NOT equal on both sides→ sinusitis).

- **UTI:** if lower (suprapubic tenderness, dysuria, frequency) order urine analysis & start abx (like bactrim or Ciprofloxacin for 3 days if uncomplicated), if upper UTI (fever, chills, CVA tenderness, dysuria) order UA & assess the need for hospital admission (elderly, multiple comorbidities, septic signs, etc) for IV abx (Ciprofloxacin or zosyn). UTI can be categorized to "uncomplicated", which is in lower UTI in female for the 1st time. The rest is complicated (male even for the 1st time, recurrence, Upper UTI, etc).

Attention: no need to follow UTI response to abx by urine analysis or urine Cx. Clinical improvement is enough (unless in pregnancy → Tx even asymptomatic bacteriuria and assure resolution w/ negative urine Cx)

Gout: Usually affects the big toe (Podagra) & other joints. NO need to confirm diagnoses by arthrocentesis (to see the monosodium urate crystals).
Clinical diagnosis is enough, unless you consider another diagnose like septic joint (WBC>2k in gout while >50k in septic joint w/ positive stain & culture).
 Tx of choice: NSAIDs (if NOT contraindicated like in CKD), then colchicine, local steroid injection, & lastly systemic steroids (like prednisone PO). **Continue allopurinol if pt was on it before the flare, but do NOT initiate it** in the acute attack (rapid up or down changes in uric acid blood levels may worsen gouty attack). Scheduled dose of daily colchicines for maintenance (not just on the acute flare) can also be prescribed in case of allopurinol allergy (should be

dosed renally). **Probenecid** (inhipit uric acid tubular reabsorption but contraindicated in CKD) & **Uloric** (like allopurinol but expensive). Target uric acid <7.

Smoke/EtOH & illicit drugs: assess for abuse in every visit & counsel to stop w/ a clear direct sentence like "this abuse will/already hurt your body & vital organs like lung, heart, liver, etc & if you stop you may stop the progression. If you are interested I can assist you". If the pt is NOT interested, you can readdress it in a later visit (spending much time in counseling if the pt is NOT interested in quitting did NOT prove to be successful). Offer nicotine patches/gum or even meds like Wellbutrin & Chantix (good for depression as well) to ↓ grieving Sx (but insurance may NOT cover them) or even referral to rehabilitation center (for EtOH & drug abuse)

Dermatology:
- **Shingles:** Reactivation of latent varicella-zoster virus (VZV) infx w/ in the sensory ganglia results in herpes zoster or "shingles". This syndrome is usually characterized by a painful, unilateral vesicular eruption in a dermatomal distribution. Early antiviral therapy (acyclovir for 1 week for age >50) can promote rapid healing of skin lesions, lessen the severity & duration of pain associated w/ acute neuritis, & reduces the incidence or severity of chronic pain.
- **Itching:** it can be from systemic disease like liver or renal disease. Allergy from new meds is a possible cause (try to stop new meds & monitor). Xerosis (dry skin) is a common cause for pruritus. Ask about excessive h & washing or may be new detergent (which can be contact dermatitis, could be treated w/ topical steroids). **Tx:** Moisturizers such as petrolatum can help the dry skin.
  Scabies: is another possible itching etiology, which usually presents w/ severe itching, often worse at night, & nondescript erythematous

papules. Family involvement strongly suggests the diagnosis.

Tx: Ivermectine PO (which can treat lice too) & /or Permethrin (Tx the family also & wash the linens).

Polypharmacy: Frequent routine review to verify need for meds & appropriate dosing is an important aspect of optimal pt (especially elderly) care.

Altered mental status is a common adverse effect to polypharmacy (mostly psychiatry & pain meds). Assess risks & benefits for meds & consider stopping any med that has the same side effect (like statins, fibrates, & Niacins which may all damage the liver). Consider stopping meds that are NOT indicated any more like prophylactic statins for very elderly pts or anticoagx for elderly w/ ↑ risk of falls (after discussing risks & benefits).

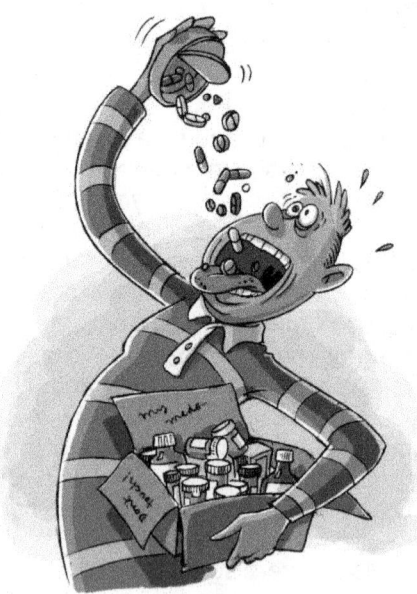

Polypharmacy is a common reason for AMS & meds interaction should be considered, especially for the elderly.

Heath Care Maintenance: In a general medicine clinic it's helpful to conclude each note w/ a health care maintenance section. This includes age & sex specific screening tests as well as vaccinations that are otherwise easy to overlook. **Common Vaccines & screening tests:**

- **PAP smear**: starting age 21-65 or 3 years after 1st sexual activity, q3 years (or q5years if PAP + HPV test). Optimal frequency is NOT established (q1-2 years is acceptable)
- **Mammogram:** females >50 usually or age 40-50 if the pt wants (usually every 1-2 years).
- **AAA screen w/ abdominal US:** male age 65-75 if ever smoker
- **Colonoscopy:** any pt >50, every 10 years (or FOBT + flex sig q5years)
- **Lung cancer screen w/ chest CT scan:** age 55-80 q1 year if >30 pack years, current smoker, or quit w/ in last 15 years (do NOT screen if quit>15 years)
- **Hyperlipidemia:** male>35 & female >45, q5 years.
- **PSA:** any male >50 (if the pt agrees but generally NOT recommended for screening w/o risks). Refer to GU for biopsy if PSA>7 (rectal exam is NOT recommended for screening)
- **DEXA scan for osteoporosis:** female >65 or <65 w/ fracture, q 2-8 years.
- **Vaccines:**
  Influenza: yearly for all adults.
  Pneumovaccines: pneumococcal polysaccharide vaccine (PPSV23), elderly>65, DM, CHF, CKD, Asthma/COPD, asplenic pts, & others.

> **Attention**: Usually screening tests are NOT recommended for pt >75 yo or pts w/ life expectancy <10 years (physician dependent).

Zoster: > 60 yo, one time (life attenuated).
Other life attenuated vaccines: Varicella, MMR, yellow fever, oral polio, & Nasal flu (most of the others are inactivated).
Tdap/Td: >19 yo, one time (but tetanus q10 yrs)
HPV vaccine: all male & female age 13-26 yo.

49. Diet & Physical/Occupational Therapy (PT/OT)

Diet: Choosing a diet is one of the tasks you will have as internal medicine resident. Remember you can always consult a nutritionist who specializes in this field for advice.

If pt is able to swallow & eat normal food then the choice of meal lies on the pt's comorbidities:
- **No significant co-morbidities** → regular diet
- **DM:** choose a diabetic, low calorie diet (<18k).
- **HTN**: low salt diet (< 2gr Na)
- **CKD/ESRD**: renal diet (low phosphate, protein & salt).
- **Cardiac**: cardiac diet (low cholesterol, low Na) diet.
- **Electrolyte abnormality:** diets can be modified (for example: hyperkalemia, you can order a low K modifier to the diet).

If a pt has **dysphagia** or is at risk for aspiration (be cautious w/ AMS & elderly pts) then a consult to speech pathology is warranted. They can perform various swallow tests from a bedside test to barium swallow study & post recommendations on what type of diet the pt could handle.

If the pt is to have a **procedure** the next day, then make sure an order is placed to be NPO at midnight. Many conditions such as pancreatitis, altered mental status, bowel obstruction require the pt to be NPO from admission until further evaluation or improvement of the condition.

Consider NOT resuming the same home insulin dose if the pt is NPO or has poor appetite. Resume the long acting & add fast acting just PRN if pt ate >80% of the meal.

Nutrition is an important part of hospitalized pts, & you will see many pts w/ chronic conditions that have malnutrition. A good marker of malnutrition is low prealbumin level.

Chronic malnutrition:
 Consider nutrition consult. They can recommend a variety of diets plus diet enhancements (such as protein shakes), & possibly appetite stimulants to help w/ the pt's nutrition status. If a pt is **chronically unable to obtain proper nourishment** after interventions, then it is appropriate to begin discussing other options of feeding such as tube feeds.
If a pt has a **poor prognosis** w/ limited life expectancy make sure talks about hospice care are initiated before beginning to discuss invasive gastric devices for supportive feedings.

Tube feedings:
It is a good idea to initiate tube feedings by the third day of hospitalization in pts who are unable to swallow (& if no contraindications exist).
Nutritionist can dose tube feedings rate but usually you start low (like 10 cc/h) of feeding fluid like high fiber/high calorie & increasing rate may be q3-6 hrs as tolerated (nurses can check stomach residual which should below in good GI motility status) w/ max rate may be 60-70cc/h.

> **Attention**: Free water flushes by NG or PEG tube (can be administered w/ the same feeding pump) is a good route to treat hypernatremia (like 250cc/3hrs for total of the amount of the free water deficit).

PEG tube (can be placed by GI or general surgery) is a good long term feeding route for pt w/ swallow difficulty, long term intubation, or any unconscious pt as NG tube is NOT recommended for more than 5-7 days.

PT/OT:

Many hospital pts become deconditioned w/ long hospital stays. Order PT/OT consults sooner rather than later. They will help the pt build strength & make recommendations on what the pt will need on discharge whether it be home PT (which is set up through the case manager), home medical equipment, or an acute rehab facility.

If the pt requires an **acute rehab facility**, it is wise to discuss this w/ the social work team early as this can delay discharge.

50. Diseases and diagnosis need high suspicion

This topic includes diagnoses, which may NOT be very clear or obvious, & need↑ level of suspicion to identify in every pt given the right circumstances.

Decubitus ulcers: mostly on the pressure points like the sacrum & heels. The main risk factor is immobility (fractures, paralysis, elderly, & critically ill). When admitting a new pt, you need to turn them to look for decubitus ulcers & document your findings. This is NOT only important for the pt, but also for payment for the hospital as newly acquired decubitus ulcers during hospital stay can result in non-payment.

Staging pressure/decubitus ulcers:
Stage I: Skin is intact w/ non-blanching redness in a localized area.
Stage II: Partial-thickness loss of dermis, which presents as a shallow open ulcer w/ a red-pink wound base.
Stage III: Full-thickness tissue loss w/ visible subcutaneous fat, however bone, tendon or muscles are NOT exposed.
Stage IV: Full-thickness tissue loss w/ exposed bone, tendon & /or muscle.

Tx: The main components you have to think about when treating a pressure ulcer are relieving or reducing the pressure, wound care w/ possible need for debridement of necrotic tissue, monitoring the bacterial load & presence of infx, & pain control.
Pressure relief w/ proper positioning & support surfaces is important, including scheduled turning of bedbound pts. Local wound care, including selecting a proper dressing is important; surgical debridement may be necessary.
Choosing a dressing depends on the stage of the ulcer, the amount of exudate being drained from the wound, presence of infx or tunneling, & the surrounding skin.

Assessing for pain control is also important in wound care, especially during dressing changes.
Non-opioid topical preparations such as lidocaine/prilocaine may reduce the pain during changes as well as repositioning. Also, look for signs of infx such as warmth, erythema, local tenderness, & purulent foul odor discharge. Optimize nutrition status.

Substance abuse: This is an important part of the H & P but the pt may NOT volunteer the information. Some drugs associated w/ common presenting Sx include the following: cocaine & CP, hallucinogens & altered mental status, alcohol & vomiting or falls. These associations need to be in the differential & can be diagnosed by complete social hx & urine drug screen. Be aware that the drug screen does NOT include all the drugs that a pt could have used like LSD & EtOH.

Pain meds: Pain is a subjective feeling, & is hard to be measured accurately. When a pt is requesting pain meds, always ask for a full hx of the pain complaints, & assess the reliability of the hx. Note unspoken cues such as face reaction on physical exam & the consistency of their reactions. Also, use objective tests like X-rays for joint pain (knee or back) & consider non-narcotic pain meds vs. narcotics. Have a high threshold to prescribe opioids for pts w/ hx of substance abuse. Oxycodone (w/o the Tylenol) has a high street value, & substance abusers can administer it by other routes besides PO, like IV & intranasal.

Meds: always think about the pt's current or past meds as a guide for differential diagnosis & even management. **For AMS:** benzodiazepines, antiemetics, or antipsychotics could contribute or be the cause of the AMS. **For acute urinary retention:** look at TCA antidepressants, 2nd G antipsychotics (Clozapine) or Benadryl as they have anti-cholinergic effects.

Non-compliance (diet or meds): It is very important to know if a pt is compliant w/ recommended diet & meds, especially for chronic conditions needing long-term therapy & diet restriction, such as CHF & ESRD. Water restriction to 1-1. 5 L of fluid & a ↓Na diet of<2 g/day are very important to prevent decompensation in those conditions. In fluid restriction, liquid foods like soups have to be taken into account. In Na-restricted diets, salty foods, including canned goods & pickles have to be restricted along w/ the use of salt in cooking.

> **Attention:** Simple pt education may prevent complications & unnecessary adjusting of meds & doses. When there is non-adherence, ask for the reason & change the meds w/ unpleasant side effects, if possible.

Wrong results: Look at the pt's presentation including the H & P & think about the test result consistency w/ the presentation. Compare the results w/ a previous one to have a helpful trend, & repeat the abnormal lab.
Example: a pt in the hospital had a stable Cr for a few days, & then had one reading which showed the Cr had doubled. Repeat the BMP before ordering a kidney US & urine electrolytes (cost effective & time saving). Or if a pt's blood pressure it too high or low, repeat the blood pressure measurement, including trying a manual measurement, before you manage, especially if the pt is asymptomatic.

51. Cost-effective medicine

Now this has become an important subject given the rise of ordering tests & the practice of defensive medicine. Given how much we spend on healthcare, what we can do as physicians to help this matter is order using a cost effective approach for our pts. This prevents unnecessary procedures & tests for our pts while still providing the same standard of care w/ a lower cost.

Example: Resident A: takes care of a 55 y/o female w/ shortness of breath w/ a cost of $20, 000. **Resident B:** takes care of the same pt & had a cost of $10, 000. Clearly, if I was a pt I would want the doctor to provide the same care w/ half the price, w/o unnecessary testing, & ↓ Length of stay. Before we go into cost effective medicine, we have to understand & use statistics as this will be our friend when determining to order CT scans, MRI, PET scans, etc.

Next are some definitions to common terminology helps in interpreting the test results & some common sense ideas help in the daily practice.
Sensitivity: ability of a test to detect disease when present
Specificity: ability of a test to exclude disease when absent
Pre-test probability: the likelihood that a pt has a specific disease before any testing
Post-test probability: the likelihood that a pt has a specific disease after a test has been done

Likelihood ratios: very useful in clinical practice based on test characteristics & prevalence data. Utilizes pretest probability of disease in a specific pt & tests sensitivity/specificity. They give us how much a given test would change our pretest probability of disease for a post probability change. The likelihood ratio of >1 indicates the test result is associated w/ the disease so higher pretest probability of the disease. A likelihood

262

ratio < 1 indicates that the result is associated w/ absence of the disease so lower pretest probability of the disease; a Likelihood ratio of 1 has no practical significance in the disease.

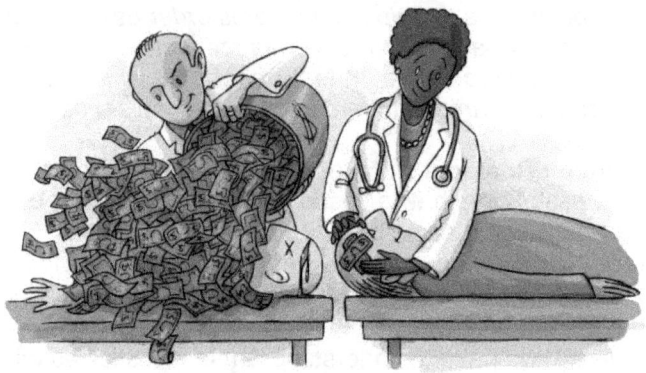

Practicing cost-effective medicine is putting the right money in the right place.

Other **pearls** & ideas for cost effective medicine:
- **Empiric abx coverage w/o indication** occurs in complicated pictures with sick pts. Assess the need for those abx in daily basis & stop them if you still do NOT have infectious etiology (especially after 2-3 days & if pt is NOT improving).

> **Attention**: Over prescribing abx w/o indication spread resistance in adition to the high cost for pts receiving abx that are NOT indicated or warranted in that particular scenario.

- **Daily labs & CXR** when it is NOT going to change the Tx plans or diagnosis are NOT needed & cause pt discomfort & even anemia in the case of lab work in the long run.

- **When you have source of infx** (like abdominal abscess) you may NOT need more than blood & pus cultures to know the organism. Pan-culture (urine, sputum & blood) is NOT needed unless it is indicated.
- **No need for CBC w/ diff** if you are following Hgb for GI bleeding. Instead just order H & H.
- **CBC w/ differential is NOT necessary if no infx suspected.** CBC w/o differential is enough.
- **Out pt records/tests can be asked for** in nonemergency situations & it saves the costs & the inconvenience for the pt from going to the same tests again.
- **Choose cheaper abx** for the same indication & coverage & switch from IV to PO as soon as indicated (especially if pt is tolerating PO & you have culture sensitivity)
- **CXR changes after PNA can stay up to 6 weeks** & a follow up x-ray may be indicated to confirm resolution (no need to repeat x ray w/ in 6 weeks unless Sx are changed)
- **Order BMP & NOT CMP** if hepatic function test is NOT needed in you assessment & plan
- **PO meds are preferred over IV meds** if there is no indication for the ladder (like dysphagia, rapid effectiveness, intestine edema like in ascites, accurate dose delivery, etc.)
- **Reassess the need of**: telemetry, Foley cath, IV fluids & abx, on a daily basis & discontinue them when indicated. You can stop empiric abx coverage (like vanc/zosyn) after 3-5 days if the pt became afebrile & no source of infx was found.
- **For pts that will need placement:** place PPD on admission & get social worker early in the process to help ↓ length of hospital stay
- **Review & reconcile meds** on admission & discharge & even in daily bases. Stop any meds that are NOT needed any more.

- **Educate pts about the length of Tx** for each meds, especially the abx & the PRN meds (like the pain & N/V meds)

Attention: to social hx & alcohol consumption. Start the pt on alcohol withdrawal protocol along w/ the necessary vitamins (thiamine), which will prevent dealing w/ hard to treat & chronic conditions like delirium tremens & Wernicke-korsakoff dementia

Attention: to health maintenance vaccine & indicated screening tests like mammography & colonoscopy can help in preventing & treating problems in early stages.

- Hospital Length Of Stay LOS can be significantly ↓ by using **"swing beds"** available in another facilities which are designed to take care patient who are NOT ready to go home but they are still needing skilled nursing care. Swing Bed is like a bridge from the hospital before going home & it gives the patient time to heal & adjust before returning to everyday life.
Examples of skilled care include:
  · IV therapy
  · Sterile dressing changes
  · Skin/wound care
  · Rehabilitation therapy: physical therapy, occupational therapy, speech therapy & respiratory therapy.

52. Refer to specialist & inpatient consultation

Refer to specialist:
- **Diabetes mellitus type I** to endocrinology, as sometimes it is hard to manage w/ the traditional insulin regimen. Pt w/ long standing DM type I (more than 10 years) or DMII should be referred to ophthalmology or nephrologist for further DM complicationsTx.
- **CKD stage 3** when glomerular filtration rate is less than 60 needs close follow up/preparation for dialysis access when needed. Usually AV fistulas need months for maturation & to be accessible.
- **New diagnoses of arrhythmia & CHF:** there are reversible causes & can be investigated w/ more invasive work up like electrophysiology lab or cardiac cath.
- **Pulmonary rehab, cardiac rehabilitation, & physical therapy** should be considered for COPD, CHF & Fibromyalgia pts, respectively. Improves quality of life (especially for end stage cases).
- **Cancer pts** (or high suspicion of malignancy) can be referred to hem/onc clinic as they best discuss Tx options & side effects along w/ the prognosis. Chemotherapy can be complicated & some of them are experimental.

In patient consultation: Make sure you mention the reason for the consult (or the question you have for the consultant) before you go into the details of the pt's medical hx (like I am consulting cardiology to help managing new onset of SVT which did NOT respond to adenosine & IV β blocker). Put on mild that we should NOT consult cardiology for each single common cardiology matter, especially if we you are managing the pt the right way & the pt is responding. Be ready to answer any question from the consultant such as lab results, vitals, radiology results, & so forth (in another word, Know your pt very well).

Examples:

- **Cardiology consultation:** form the consult as a question you want their help in answering it after at least trying a common interevention (especially in non-urgent situation). You should check for recent TTE (EF? Or valvular disease?), EKG (ischemic changes?), stress test (CAD?), heart caths, cardiac enzymes, PMH (especially cardiac hx like CAD, arrhythmias, HTN, DM, Valvular disease, etc), pacemaker/ICD devices. Baseline exercise tolerance is important to know for any cardiac complaints or preoperational risk stratification (walk for 1 mile/climb 2 flights of stairs w/o SOB?). Certain problems needs an urgent/emergent consults like STEMI

- **GI consult:** you should check for previous EGD/colonoscopy w/ results for any GI bleed, Abdominal US, ERCP, bilirubin, Alkphos, liver enzymes for any biliary tract problem, & amylase & lipase for pancreatic problem. Unstable GI bleeding may need an urgent consult for possible scope (while resuscitating & stabilize the pt).

- **Nephrology consult**: you should check for Cr (current & baseline in the last few weeks/months), BUN, urine electrolytes (for AKI), BMP (calculate the gap if academic), volume status, dialysis access (if the pt on dialysis).

- **Neurology consult:** you should know recent MRIs, CTs, carotid doppler, TTE, & baseline neuro function for stroke pts. Know the duration, description, meds, glucose, & electrolyte levels for seizure pts

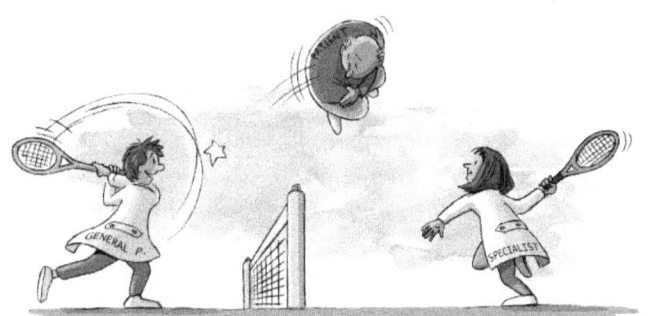

Referral at the right time is part of practicing optimal medicine.

53. Common unclear diagnoses

Some diagnoses or Sx are NOT the presenting problem & the pt does NOT complain from them specifically, but they are affecting other common Sx or diseases. Think about these etiologies in every pt. Some examples:

- **Morbid obesity**: BMI >40 (or even obesity w/ BMI 30-40) has a strong association w/o OSA, Obesity Hypoventilation Syndrome OHS (elevated Co2), musculoskeletal pains (back pain & chest pain,especially w/ extremely large breasts), early osteoarthritis (OA), Congestive heart failure (diastolic & systolic), LVH, cardiac arrhythmias, & metabolic syndrome ($\uparrow$ blood sugar, high BP, dyslipidemia). Finding the relationship between those diagnoses & the obesity is essential to properly manage the pt. Address the obesity early enough by diet/exercise or even more aggressively by bariatric surgery referral (for possible bypass or gastric band) may make the medical therapy more effective or even unnecessary.
- **Dilutional anemia:** is common in pregnancy as the plasma $\uparrow$ to reach 50% & RBCs $\uparrow$ to 30% (usually if the anemia is less than 10. 5, another diagnosis should be sought). Excessive IV fluid effusion can cause dilutional effect as well. Look at the other 2 lines of blood, the WBC & platelets. If they are $\downarrow$ at the same % then the etiology may be dilutional.
- **Irritable bowel syndrome**: Abdominal pain at least 3 times/month for the last 3 months w/ improvement w/ defecation & change in stool appearance & frequency. Make sure there are no alarming Sx like: iron deficiency anemia, GI bleeding, weight loss, nocturnal Sx & family hx of colon ca, IBD, & celiac disease. Tx:

Symptomatic (laxatives for constipation & anti spasmatics for diarrhea), antidepressants, or referral to GI.

- **Fibromyalgia**: Pain & tenderness in 11/18 points along w/ fatigue & difficulty sleeping. Keep work-up to a minimum such as CBC & ESR (for inflammation or infx). Best Tx is exercise & rehab programs. Use meds as a 2nd line (SNRI like duloxetine or TCA like amitriptyline).
- **Anxiety**: Generalized worry, irritability, fatigue, body pain, SOB, & sleep disturbance (usually it is the 1st to resolve after Tx). Management: Cognitive & behavioral therapy CBT (try to identify the stressor & distinguish if it is from an extrinsic source like divorce or recent death or if it is intrinsic) & medical Tx (like Lexapro, paroxetine, sertraline, & imipramine). Weigh the risks & benefits for benzodiazipins. Sometimes you need to ask specifically about anxiety if the pt is complaining about many Sx which are NOT connected.

Attention: Mental health diagnoses like somatization & malingering disorders → needs high suspicion to recognize and Tx.

- **Obstructive sleep apnea (OSA)**: Very common (20-30% male & 10-15% female) & needs high suspicion to elicit the diagnosis. More common in obese population but also present in pts w/ normal BMI. **Symptoms:** excessive fatigue during the day, possible right heart failure signs & Sx along w/ pulm HTN, systemic HTN, depression, poor concentration, continuous moving (to stay awake but fall a sleep when reading a book or newspaper), cardiac conduction problems (like a fib) & morning HA. Ask the pt or a family member such as the spouse if the pt snores, has apneas, or wakes up at night gasping for air as if pt was choking. **Diagnose** w/ sleep study & **treat** w/ C-PAP mainly (needs ↑compliance as it is uncomfortable to use so always ask about compliance). PO appliance & surgery are also options (but C-PAP is the best Tx).

- **Acute abdominal angina (acute mesenteric ischemia)**: Etiology: most common is embolism from somewhere else. Atherosclerosis w/ ↓ perfusion (like in sepsis or HoTN) or artery/venous thrombosis can cause the ischemic pain. Look for pain out of proportion to the abdominal tenderness, N/V, lower GI bleed, & severe pain w/ negative tests such as normal abdominal US & x-ray (CTA is the test of choice). Check lactic acid & consult surgery for possible resection if the intestine is inviable.

- **Meds incompliance/incorrect use**: Thyroxine should be taken in the morning 30 minutes before the 1st meal. Follow up w/ TSH 6-8 weeks after adjusting thyroxine dose & make sure that the pt is taking the thyroxine as scheduled on an empty stomach before adjusting the dose. CPAP is very uncomfortable to use & adherence need to be assessed in regular bases. Low Na diet & water restriction need to be assessed with CHF, HTN & ESRD pts on HD.

- **COPD/asthma inhalations**: Counsel the pt to exhale all the way & then inhale the puffs all the way & wait for few seconds. A "spacer" is an option for the children or elderly who do NOT inhale the right way. Educate about the "rescue" inhaler such as the albuterol which is used just as needed for wheezing & SOB, & the "scheduled" inhaler which should be taken ALL the time as scheduled even w/ no Sx.

- **β blocker & statins side effects**: Ask about the side effects of the meds when you suspect incompliance. β blockers can cause orthostatic HoTN & impotence & the pt may just stop taking them. Statins may also cause flu like Sx & myopathies. Asking about these side effect can help you determine the right management which may be involve decreasing the doses or switch to another med w/ less problems.
- **Insulin skips & diet incompliance:** Diabetes is a life-long disease, especially for type I, requires a↑ degree of compliance w/ the insulin & the diet. Pts may present w/ hypoglycemia if they took full dose of insulin & they did NOT eat full meal or delayed the meal (especially important for fast acting insulin like aspart. Refer to diabetic diet educator as needed.
- **Depression**: Screen when appropriate w/ **2 Qs:** Over the past 2 weeks, have you felt down, depressed & hopeless? Have you felt little pleasure or interests in doing things you were previously interested in?
  If yes, ask the rest of the depression Qs. Assess suicidal ideations & plans. Treat w/ antidepressants if it is a1st time, NOT complicated diagnosis.

  Refer to psychiatry if it is recurrent, NOT responding to the first Tx trial, if complex comorbidities exist, & in the presence of suicidal ideations (may need to go to the ED for that). **Choose the antidepressants** based on the side effect profile & comorbidities. Commonly used ones: Celexa (citalopram), Prozac (fluoxetine), Paxil (paroxetine), Zoloft (sertraline), Effexor (venlafaxine), Pristiq (desvenlafaxine), Cymbalta (duloxetine), trazodone, Wellbutrin (buproption, used for smoking cessation, lowers threshold for seizures). **Assess side effects** after 2 weeks of

Tx & the **response of Tx** & improvement in mood after 6-8 weeks.

Monitor pts carefully after Tx, especially in adolescents & young adults, & ask about suicidal thoughts & plans (as they have more energy to suicide after Tx). Psychotherapy is a good option to consider along w/ the meds. Add 2nd depression med if the pt responded partially to Tx like sleeping better after the 1st med but he/she still feels depressed & hopeless.

Attention: Insomnia & sleep disturbance is the 1st Sx to respond to depression Tx & is a good indicator to follow after starting the meds.

- **Adrenal cortical suppression ($\downarrow$ cortisol)**:
  Etiology: iatrogenic (from chronic steroid Tx like in COPD & immune diseases like SLE & rheumatoid arthritis), Addison's disease (adrenal cortical atrophy, $\uparrow$ ACTH), central (pituitary problem, $\downarrow$ ATCH, mineral hormone like aldosterone is still intact cause of the rennin/angiotensin axis), or cancer.

  General signs: cachexia, anorexia, weight loss, hypercalcemia, bone pain, & metastasis effects. Specific signs: SOB (pulmonary effect), AMS (brain mets), etc. A high level of suspicion is required as the Sx are very nonspecific.

  Diagnose w/ $\downarrow$ cortisol (order the test early in the morning as the level fluctuates normally during the day. You can order random cortisone levels but it needs to be very $\downarrow$ to be diagnostic). ACTH stimulation test is a good diagnostic test (measure baseline cortisol & give ACTH like med- Cosynotropin, repeat cortisol check in 30m & 60m & assess the response).

Tx: high dose IV hydrocortisone (better than other steroid forms). Stressors like infx & surgery will need additional doses of steroids for pts who are chronically taking them.

- **Influenza**: pulmonary Sx like cough, rhinorrhea, fever, pleuretic pain, & fatigue; r/o influenza w/ easy A & B flu swab tests. Try NOT to lose the 2 dayTx window of anti-flu meds like oseltamivir (Tamiflu) as it is most effective in the 1st 48h window after the appearance of Sx.
- **Osteoporosis** is common disease & can be screened for (postmenopausal, pts w/ risk factors, or age >65) w/ a DEXA scan.
  Tx: Aldronate or risedronate along w/ Vitamin D, Ca^{2+}, & weight-baring exercise. Diagnosis & Tx of osteoporosis can prevent a very debilitating hip or other bone fracture, especially in the elderly.

54. Different approaches for common problems

Sometime, Sx & diagnoses are NOT very clear or straightforward. The following are common ideas to consider in approaching some common diagnoses.

- **HTN** may be due to pain, bladder fullness, volume overload, extensive IV fluid, DT from alcohol withdrawal, White coat phobia, rebound HTN from stopping hypotensive meds like β blockers, or substance abuse or withdrawal such as from cocaine or heroin. Treat the cause of the HTN, NOT just the numbers.
- **Mental health pts**: like schizophrenia, depression/anxiety, or fibromyalgia can have serious problems as well & their complaints should be taken seriously & ruled out appropriately as indicated.
- **TSH abnormality:** do NOT change the thyroxine dose before making sure that the pt is taking the meds on empty stomach & during the daytime. TSH can be abnormal in an in pt setting due to sick thyroid, & it is more accurate to adjust the thyroxine dose in out pt setting. Consider following TSH levels 4-6 weeks after adjusting the thyroxine dose. ↑ Thyroixine dose in pregnancy by 30% (as thyroxine binding protein normally ↑)
- **Repeat the tests:** that you suspect are wrong or inconsistent before ordering other costly follow up tests or changing your care plan. **Examples:** repeat the test if you see ↑ serum Cr in few of your pts at the same time w/ no clear reason, or if your pt has a low Hgb compared to their baseline w/ no signs or Sx of bleeding.
- **Thiamine IV:** should be given to pts w/ chronic alcoholism to prevent Wernicke-Korsakoff syndrome (signs are fabrication, nystagmus, &

abnormal finger nose sign or ataxia). Have a low threshold to put the pts on vitamins & SIWA protocol if they present w/ altered mental status & hx of falls, causing you to consider alcohol abuse. Sometimes, calling the family is very informative in recognizing a pt's alcohol abuse hx.

- **Order the tests that may be useful:** in working through your differential diagnosis & that may help you w/ further management. Abnormal or borderline values can be difficult to interpret if they are NOT obtained in the right scenario & if there is low pretest probability. Think about practicing cost effective medicine.
- **Science of simplicity:** when you encounter new pt & after finishing all the important pt's details & formulating the plan, approaching that pt again, briefly, can make the pt more memorable (especially in a busy day).

Attention: "The science of simplicity" is applied in medicine as most of our pts population has 5-10 problems (even up to 25) & sometimes you will have up to 10-20 new patient/day.

The following may be enough to remember & recognize the pt: pt's name, chief complaint, diagnosis (or top 3 differentials), abnormal tests (may be done in the ED or in another hospital), important tests you ordered, pt's status (stable or critical which may need more than one visit/day), & expected discharge date. In essence, don't sweat the small stuff. Make it easier by concentrating on the big picture. Correspondingly, a number of very successful doctors have adopted this philosophy in their daily routines.

For example: if pt is admitted for PNA; know the CXR, WBC, fever, SOB status, cultures, abx, hydration status, & responding to Tx so you know when to discharge. Focusing on electrolytes abnormalities, elevating CBG if diabetic, BP elevation if hypertensive, feeling nauseated, low appetite, & other side Sx may NOT need to be at the top of your head (of course remembering the essentials & the details is great & encouraged but this approach is a plan B to avoid remembering the details & losing the whole picture).

55. Social support & social history

The social hx is an important part of the H & P to help you know the pt, formulate a better differential diagnosis, & more efficient discharge planning. Ask about accommodations, who lives w/ the pt & helps him/her w/ meds & medical care, marriage status & children, habits (tobacco, EtOH & illicit drug use), work status & sexual hx.

a. **Elderly:** Assess the ability of the pt to return home if the pt is living alone & make early arrangements for appropriate placement w/ a social worker. It is best to start working on this on the day of admission as this part of discharge planning can take a great deal of time & lead to unnecessary days in the hospital. Assess the risk of falls & make the pt's family aware of the need for assistance & physical therapy. Assisted living or nursing home placement should be discussed if the pt's family canNOT meet the pt's new needs of care, & again, this topic needs to be approached early in the hospital course.

b. **Smoking:** You have to ask how much & for how long. Smoking is a direct risk factor for many diseases such as COPD, CAD, cancers, & PAD. Ask the pt if he/she is interested in quitting. If yes, you can offer meds to ↓ the nicotine withdrawal Sx like nicotine replacement (patches or gum), Chantix (nicotine agonist), & bupropion (Wellbutrin, an antidepressant). If not, tell them in short sentences that smoking is bad for their health & you are available to help when they are ready to quit. When a pt is NOT ready to quit, extensive talking & brochures have NOT shown any benefit in quitting.

c. **Alcohol:** ask CAGE Questions: Have you thought about **C**utting down? Have you ever gotten **A**nnoyed when people talk to you about your drinking? Have you ever felt **G**uilty about your drinking? Do you ever have a drink first thing in the morning (**E**ye opener)? If two or more are positive the pt has EtOH dependency, & may need EtOH withdrawal prophylaxis (CIWA protocol) w/ Ativan to prevent delirium tremens (DTs).

DTs manifest as hallucinations, disorientation, tachycardia, HTN, fever, agitation, & diaphoresis & have ↑ mortality rate. **History:** focus on how much drinks, kind, for how long, did pt ever quite (looking for previous DT), is pt willing to quite now, any rehap was tried, any family support (wife or kids), & mental status to r/o wernicke-korsakoff.

The main Tx for alcohol withdrawal, including Delirium Tremens DTs, is benzodiazepines w/ Ativan IV or PO being the most commonly used. You can give as much as needed to control the Sx & the vitals. Replete vitamins whenever admitting a pt dependent on alcohol, especially thiamine IV or PO (in addition to other vitamins included in banana bag), to prevent Wernicke-Korsakoff syndrome. **Librium (taper dose):** is a long acting benzos (less Euphoria effect) which can be used to continue preventing DTs as an out pt.

Alcohol abstinence is part of the transplantation criteria for liver (abstinence for 6months)/Kidney (3 months)/heart transplant (3 months) & it should be documented by a physician. Consider ordering Gama-glutamyl transferase (GGT) in recent EtOH intake as well as blood EtOH levels & AST (↑ more than ALT).

> **Attention:** It is unknown how much is too much of EtOH to cause permanent liver or heart disease due to different metabolisms. Usually it is caused from a minimum use of 6-7 beers a day (or equivalent) for >6-7 years (or any amount with end organ damage)

d. **Physical therapy:** PT is ordered when there is a concern about the pt's safety & based on observations while in hospital. Assess the need for in pt vs. out pt PT for the appropriate pts who have balance problems, hx of falls, after surgeries, & for the elderly. Also, PT can evaluate & recommend ambulating assistance devices like walkers & wheelchairs & necessary placement, such as subacute rehab, acute rehab, & a skilled nursing facility, as indicated. **Occupational therapy** helps to achieve independence & improve one's ability to perform daily activities & self-care. It is usually needed w/ the physical therapy, especially for elderly.

e. **Home health:** Home health can provide skilled nurses part-time or on an intermittent basis to help in out pt settings. Services they can provide include meds administration (even IV meds), out pt PT/OT, wound care (dressing changes), & tube feeding.

f. **Medical consent for procedure:** Consent is an important part of procedures & it will save a lot of time if the procedure is predicted & the consent was taken early in the admission when the family was available, especially for pts w/ dementia or unable to consent. **Phone consent** is an option & you can try to take a phone number from the pt's caregiver at the time of admission. For consent you should explain the pros & cons for the procedure in an understandable fashion. An emergency procedure does NOT need consent, although it is recommended to take a minute to call the family & document that in the records.

56. Incidental findings & mildly abnormal tests

Tests sometimes show incidental abnormalities, which need to be followed up. Sometimes abnormal findings may be age related, NOT severe enough to cause a problem or mild & do NOT need to be followed very closely.

*Here are some **examples**:*

- **Solitary Pulmonary nodules:** a solitary pulm nodule (SPN) is a lesion that is surrounded by normal pulm parenchyma w/ no additional alarming signs (like hilar adenopathy, atelectasis, or pleural effusion), mostly seen on CXR or computed tomography (CT) scan. Noncontrast, thin slice CT of the chest provides the optimal evaluation of nodule characteristics. When available, old imaging studies including chest radiograph & /or CT should be reviewed to determine stability or growth (it is reassuring if the lesion is the same size or smaller). The most common causes are benign including infectious granulomas & hamartomas.
  Follow up CT scans are recommended to ensure stability (usually up to 2 years w/ varying intervals depending on the nodule characteristics).
  Refer to CT surgery for possible resection or biopsy in the case of growth or in high-risk pts (smokers or cancer pts).
- **Thyroid nodule:** discovered either by palpation or incidentally noted on a radiologic study, such as carotid ultrasonography, neck CT, etc. Thyroid scintigraphy should be performed in pts w/ a ↓ serum TSH concentration.
  Fine needle aspiration (FNA) biopsy is the most accurate method for evaluating thyroid nodules (mostly for cold nodules as hot nodules

are rarely malignant) & selecting pts for thyroid surgery.

Work up: thyroid function tests, Iodine scan to determine the function & distinguish if it is "cold" or "hot" & refer to endocrinology or ENT (especially if it is cold).

- **Adnexal mass/Ovarian cyst:** common gynecologic problem that may be found in females of all ages. Some pts w/ an adnexal mass present w/ Sx or findings on physical examination. Pelvic pain or pressure is the most common Sx of an adnexal mass. Other potential Sx or signs include abnormal genital tract bleeding, abdominal distension, ascites, & hirsutism.

Many adnexal masses are asymptomatic, & the mass is discovered as an incidental finding on pelvic imaging. Features that are suggestive of malignancy include a solid mass that is irregular, fixed, or associated w/ posterior cul-de-sac nodularity. Pelvic ultrasound is the 1st line imaging study for the evaluation of an adnexal mass.

> **Attention**: conisder pregnancy test or malignancy in ovarian cysts depending on the risk factors & signs (Family hx, age, lymphoadenopathy, etc.). Refer to gynecology for further evaluation.

- **Breast mass or cyst:**
For Masses: The clinical presentation of a palpable breast mass is variable. The characteristics of the mass that need to be evaluated include density (soft, hard, firm), skin changes, nipple/areolar changes, & fixation to the chest wall. Imaging studies of a breast mass include mammography, which depicts a mass as a soft tissue density w/ sharp or spiculated

margins. An ultrasound documents if the mass is solid or cystic as well as the character of the margins & the presence of a blood supply (mammogram is NOT a good modality to test dense breast tissue in women <40 yo). Breast masses in young women (< 30 yo) that are clinically consistent w/ a benign lesion such as a fibroadenoma & in whom there is no family hx of breast cancer can be first imaged by ultrasound. The **definitive diagnosis** of a breast mass is made by a breast biopsy, which includes fine needle aspiration, core biopsy, or open biopsy. Core biopsy is preferred, which provides sufficient tissue for differentiation between invasive & noninvasive cancers as well as for hormone receptor analysis.

For cysts: Breast cysts are fluid-filled. They can present w/ Symptomatic gross palpable masses or as microcysts, usually found as an abnormality on imaging. Pts generally seek medical attention for palpable masses or associated discomfort. Simple cysts, clustered microcysts, & cysts w/ thin septa are considered benign, & no intervention is needed. Fine needle aspiration (FNA) can be performed if the cyst is Symptomatic (painful) or obscures adjacent breast tissue.

- **CT head:** CT head is usually done when looking for intra-cranial processes like bleeding, acute ischemic changes (which take 2-3 days to show in CT scan), SAH, signs of infx or tumor (which show better w/ contrast), & midline shifting etc. Microvascular changes & mild cortical atrophy in elderly pts are age appropriate changes & may NOT indicate the need for any Tx. Sometimes you may also find sub-acute to chronic CVA ischemic changes (NOT candidate for revascularization).
- **Kidney US:** usually looks for obstruction (ureteral dilation or a stone shadow),

hydropnephrosis (moderate to severe), abscesses, etc. Mild cortical atrophy or mild hydronephrosis may NOT indicate much, especially if the scenario is NOT fitting.

- **Cholelithiasis:** asymptomatic cholelithiasis is a common disease & has a benign course (common incidental finding on ultrasound & ct scan); it does NOT need surgery unless it is symptomatic.

- **CAD:** <30% stenosis in any coronary arteries indicates CAD & may simply require optimization of risk factors (weight reduction, exercise, HTN control, lipid control, statins, & ASA). Stents are usually indicated if stenosis is >70% (stenting less than this has NOT been shown to ↓ morbidity or mortality from CAD).

- **TTE:** trace or mild valvular regurgitation or stenosis in the elderly may NOT need more than yearly TTE monitoring for progression & good teeth hygiene (to prevent infx endocarditis). The heart compensate better for regurgitation than for stenosis. Mild pulm HTN (around 30s) may indicate good management of the initial pulm HTN cause, which may include OSA, left ventricular dysfunction, mitral stenosis, etc.

- **Positive bacterial cultures:** sometimes do NOT need Tx. One out of four blood Cx is mostly contamination, especially if it is GPC. Gram- bacteria in chronic Foley cath or cystostomy (like after bladder cancer resection) pts may indicate colonization, even if UA showed WBC, & do NOT need abx (unless Symptomatic or signs of systemic infx are present such as elevated WBC & fever). Some PO flora like Gram+ bacteria may grow in sputum Cx if the specimen was obtained well (mostly saliva).

- **Spine CT & MRI:** the degree of disk degenerative disease (DDD) & spinal spurs may NOT correlate w/ the neurological Sx. The radiology changes may be severe in an asymptomatic or mildly Symptomaticpt, & vice versa. Imaging is helpful for surgical evaluation if the pt is refractory to conservative back pain management (pain meds mostly).

- **CXR:** usually the initial radiological testing for chest pathology. Atelectesis is commonly seen & may NOT need further testing as it can be an indicator of shallow breathing or from lying in bed (can be confused w/ PNA infiltrations; always correlate w/ clinical picture). Abnormal findings are generally followed by CT scan. Lung nodules are best assessed w/ CT scan (as above). Thoracentesis is NOT necessary in pts who develop small (<1 cm) pleural effusions associated w/ heart failure, PNA, or after heart surgery.

57. Medical futility

There are certain disease states that are simply too late/advanced to treat. This is an undeniable fact. Recognizing these disease states will make you a better & more efficient physician & will allow you to provide your pts w/ a reasonable & realistic plan of care no matter how sick they are. There are innumerable cases where medical Tx may be considered futile. However, application of the above-mentioned paradigm makes it easier to decide when a plan is medically futile.

Common cases that are too late to treat (or simply end stage)

Case	Realistic plan of care
Severe chronic osteomyelitis in the diabetic pt or ESRD on dialysis which both usually have diffuse atherosclerosis & blood perfusion impairment	Obtain an MRI & vascular surgery evaluation for possible surgical amputation (abx usually fails, especially if it fails once before)
ACS w/ q wave apparent on EKG	Reperfusion attempt w/ thrombolytics is too late as Q wave is a sign of a dead tissue. PCI is indicated (NOT emergent, no need to activate cath lab in the middle of the night for ACS w/ q wave in EKG), treat w/ heparin drip & other ACS medical management. Plan to reduce further ischemia by reducing all risk factors, mainly HLD, HTN, & DM
CVA w/ Sx present for 3 or more hrs	Thrombolytics are NOT indicated. Start on ASA,

	Statins & get neurology onboard.
HA, photophobia & phonophobia, along w/ mental status changes in leukemic pts	Consider CNS metastasis, perform LP to r/o infectious cause, & discuss risks & benefits of intrathecal chemotherapy sooner rather than later (poor prognosis, survival <3months w/ Tx)
bilateral recurrent pulmonary emboli in oncology pts	Consider palliative care for comfort (hyper -Coagx status in malignancy may NOT response to Tx)
CNS metastasis from any primary source, median survival of 3 months w/ a range of 0-1 year depending upon pt's age & rate of metastasis	Consider palliative care for comfort (unless it is a single metastasis & amenable to resection by neurosurgery). Whole brain radiation & GAMA knife is an option.
Sx of or confirmed diagnosis of influenza for 2 or more days	No indication for Tamiflu (too late to be effective)
Acute change in mental status & neurological findings w/ multiple cerebral infarcts of unknown date	Consider palliative care
Status post pulseless code blue & NOT gaining meaningful communication for >3-4 days (especially if seizures on EEG or brain ischemic changes in CT scan/MRI are present)	Very unlikely to get better & having purposeful communication or function. Treat seizures if present (dilantin/benzos/Keppra) & consider DNR (educate family about the prognosis & palliative care). Use therapeutic hypothermia at the next 3-4 days after the code, if available.

288

Severe COPD w/ maximized medical Tx (inhalers, steroids, home O$_2$, Vaccines & adjunctive therapy) w/ existing Sx of SOB & desaturation	May need hospital admission for nebulizer Tx & IV abx for possible infx. Consider pulmonary consult to r/o possible reversible cause & consider Palliative/hospice consult.
Severe CHF w/ maximized medical Tx (β blocker, ACEi, diuresis, Hydralazine & dinitrate, sprinolactone) w/ no reversible cause for decompensation (like elevated BP, a fib or other reversible arrhythmias, Valvular problem, etc).	Consider Milrinon drip after RHC to assess dynamics & Cardiac Index CI (may relieve Sx but no mortality benefits.) Consider also left ventricular assistant therapy LVAT (just special cardiology centers have this Tx) or heart transplant as indicated.
Disease Screening & preventive medicine (like vaccines & lipids control) in geriatric pts (especially very elderly >80-85yo)	Quality of life is important for this population & positive screening may NOT indicate intervention due to ↑ risk surgery & ↑ % of mortality from another reason. De-escalate meds therapy due to polypharmacy effect ↑ risk of ADR.
Suboptimal HTN & DM management in elderly (Hgb A1c >7 & systolic BP 140s-150s)	Less aggressive control is recommended especially if Pts have HoTN/Hypoglycemia Sx. Acceptable target A1c 7-8 & de-escalate BP meds to target BP 150s systolic.

58. Cascade of actions for common problems

Common diagnosis or lab results abnormalities sometime should trigger a cascade of actions, which are like reflexes to those abnormalities. Memorizing those actions will minimize mistakes & save time in busy service. Following are some examples:

- **Electrolytes abnormalities:**
  Like hypernatremia for instance; should trigger
  1. Find the reason (like hypovolemia from ↓ PO intake)
  2. Intervene (like starting IV normal saline, encourage PO intake or start NJ tube/PEG tube free water flushes).

> **Attention:** to calculate how much fluid you are giving depends on the free water deficits (try to put the # of the liters you are giving in the order so you do NOT forget the fluid running)

  3. Follow up w/ your intervention: like schedule BMP q 4 hrs to make sure that you intervention is working & NOT over correcting or correcting too fast (if so, ↓ the rate of the fluid)
- **Hypothrombocytopenia:** ↓ in platelets more than 50% in 24 hrs after starting any type of heparin.
  1. Suspect HIT syndrome
  2. Stop heparin
  3. Send for HIT antibodies
  4. Start Argatroban (direct Xa factor inhibitor) & watch for thrombotic events (although there is ↓ platelets but w/ HIT syndrome there is ↑ risk for thrombosis)
  5. Ask nursing to NOT flush any IV line w/ heparin (write a note on the pt's door)

6. Stop Argatroban if HIT antibodies is negative

- **Chest pain:** consider EKG, troponin (q6 hrs for 3 times), CXR, ABG, O_2, heparin drip, NTG, morphine, CTA or cardiology consult.
Choose what's appropriate depends on the exam to r/o critical conditions like ACS, pulmonary embolism & pneumothorax. Use you clinical judgment & do NOT overshot w/ all those previous intervention if ACS was just ruled out recently, clear other reason for CP like PNA, obvious chest tenderness w/ recent trauma or low suspicion for those conditions (young age w/ no comorbidities & psychiatric hx).

- **GI bleeding:**
1. Check vitals including orthostatic BP
2. Establish 2 large bore IV lines & start fluids resuscitation
3. Start pantoprazole drip (in case the bleeding is from the stomach)
4. Call GI for EGD or colonoscopy as appropriate
5. Get CBC & schedule q4-6 hrs H & H to assess for ongoing bleeding

- **Fever (or any infectious sign):**
1. Localize the infx site (cough/SOB→ PNA, urinary Sx→ UTI, chills/looking sick→ any infx including bacteremia, abdominal pain→ cholecystitis, appendicitis, diverticulitis or other abdominal infx)
2. Send for culture as appropriate (send all cultures like urine, blood, sputum if no clear infx site)
3. Get CBC w/ differentials to look for WBC & bands
4. Start empirical abx (like Vanc & zosyn) as appropriate along w/ fluid IV
5. Consider MICU evaluation for very sick pts (especially pts w/ ↑ SIRS score & shock pts w/ ↓ BP who did NOT response to 2-3 liters of IV NS)

6. Consider life-threatening infx like meningitis if you have AMS or physical exam finding suggesting it like HAs, neurological deficits or nuchal rigidity

7. Consider sliding scale insulin in addition to smaller than usual scheduled insulin dose: as infx will ↑ blood glucose but pt will have low appetite.

- **Unresponsiveness:** ACLS has the best algorithm to follow (**available online**). For pt w/ normal vitals but has ↓ level of consciousness:

  1. Check CBG (especially for diabetics on insulin) & give 50% dextrose amp if CBG is ↓.

  2. Check a recent medicine intake like morphine or benzodiazepines & give naloxone (you should see an immediate response if it is the reason for the AMS)

  3. Check urine drug screen as appropriate

  4. Consider CNS etiology like CVA or meningitis & get CT scan or lumbar puncture.

- **Death:**

  1. Check response to painful stimulas (sternal rub), **pulse** (check heart mintor, if available), **breathing sounds** (for like 1-2 minutes), **pupils reaction to light** at the bedside (& the general appearance like pale, cold & loss of muscle strength)

  2. Pronounce the death (military time) & offer condolences & empathy w/ the family

  3. Ask family when it is appropriate about organ donations (even if the pt is NOT qualified just for the paper work), autopsy to know the exact death reason; need to call the chaplain & if they need help in funeral home arrangement.

  4. Proceed w/ the paper work. You will need to list the most appropriate reason for death (like infx, sepsis, PNA, cancer, heart failure & so forth). Cardio respiratory failure by itself is NOT enough to be the only reason for death (as everybody die eventually from that reason).

- **Placement:** pts who are NOT able to live by themselves any more, for different reasons, will need placement plan early enough in order to ↓ length of hospital stay. Lack of family support, different chronic medical diseases which needs constant care, mobility problems from old age or balance issues/orthopedic problems/CVAs, dementia, etc can all necessitate subacute rehabilitation or nursing home placement (w/ social workers help).
  1. Get PT/OT evaluation: to known where is the placement in: acute/subacute rehap or nursing home depends on their level of independability.
  2. Get PPD (must of nursing homes requires it)
  3. Ask the pt (or his/her family) about placement: as they need to agree on the placement plan. If they want to get the pt home no matter what, no need to start the process.
  4. Check the pt's insurance if it will cover the expenses
  5. Check the need for long-term IV meds like abx, what kind, O_2 need & feeding tube need, as they are all should be included in the application.
  6. Assure the need for transportation at the time of pt's discharge & check w/ the social worker if the hospital can arrange for one so you don't unnecessarily keep the pt for extra days in the hospital for just transportation.

Abbreviations

Term	Abbr.
Increase	↑
decrease	↓
Acute kidney injury	AKI
Alcohol	EtOH
and	&
Arterial blood gas	ABG
Atrial fibrillation	A fib
Biopsy	bx
Bone marrow	BM
Capillary blood glucose	CBG
Cardiovascular	CV
Chest pain	CP
Chest x-ray	CXR
Congestive heart failure	CHF
Coronary artery bypass surgery	CABG
Coronary artery disease	CAD
Culture	Cx
Diabetes mellitus	DM
diabetic ketoacidosis	DKA
Differential diagnosis	DDx
Dysfunction	Dysfx
Ejection fraction	EF
Electrocardiogram	EKG
End stage renal disease	ESRD

Term	Abbr.
Esophagus gastric duodenum	EGD
Headache	HA
Hemoglobin	Hgb
History	hx
Hyperosmolar hyperglycemic nonketotic syndrome	HHNS
Hypertension	HTN
Hypotension	HoTN
Herpes Zoster Virus	HZV
Infection	Infx
Intravenous	IV
Magnesium	Mg
Medical	MICU
Medication	meds
Myocardial infarction	MI
Nausea & vomiting	N/V
Nitroglycerin	NTG
Non ST elevation myocardial Infarction	NSTE MI
Oral	PO
patient	pt
Pneumonia	PNA
Pulmonary	Pulm
Reticulocyte index	RI
Serum creatinine	Cr

ST elevation myocardial Infarction	STEMI
Symptoms Sx	Sx
Treatment Tx	Tx
Urinary tract infection	UTI
Urine analysis	UA
Urine drug screen	UDS
Vacomycin	Vanc
With	w/
With out	w/o
beta blocker	B blocker
Mean artery pressure	MAP
Cardiac output	CO
Total peripheral resistance	TPR
Heart rate	HR
Stroke volume	SV
As needed	PRN
Left bundle branch block	LBBB
Right bundle branch block	RBBB
Aspirin	ASA
Gastroenterolo-gy	GI
CT angiography	CTA
Arterial blood gas	ABG
Deep venous thrombosis	DVT
Tissue Plasminogen	tPA
Jogular venous	JVD

distension	
Right ventricle	RV
Brain natriuretic peptide	BNP
Basic metabolic panel	BMP
Rapid plasma reagin	RPR
Infective endocarditis	IE
Anti nuclear antibodies	ANA
Anti-neutrophil cytoplasmic antibody	ANCA
Fecal occult blood test	FOBT
peripherally inserted central catheter	PICC line
Small bowel obstruction	SBO
Community acquired pneumonia	CAP
Healthcare acquired pneumonia	HCAP
Ventricular fibrillation	VF
Gram positive/negativ e	G+/-
Proton pumb inhipitor	PPI
Over the counter	OTC
Atriovenous malformation	AVM
Central nervous system	CNS
Cerebral vascular disease	CVA
Levt ventricular assist device	LVAT
Left anterior descending	LAD

Right coronary artery	RCA
Creatine phosphokinase	CPK
Patent foramen ovale	PFO
Drug-eluting stent	DES
partial pressure arterial oxygen	PaO2
fraction of inspired oxygen	FiO2
Acute respiratory distress syndrome	ARDS
glomerular basement membrane	GBM
Primary care provider	PCP
Benign prostatic hyperplasia	BPH
Non-invasive positive pressure ventilation	NIPPV or NIV
Fresh frozen plasma	FFP

Hydrochlorothiazide	HCTZ
Calcium channel blocker	CCB
Drug adverse effect	DAE
Pulmonary function test	PFT
Hemodialysis	HD
Hemoglobin	Hgb
Ventilation/perfusion	V/Q
Esophagogastroduodenoscopy	EGD
Transthoracic Echocardiogram	TTE
Dyspnia on exertion	DOE
Percutaneous coronary angiogram/intervention	PCA/ PCI
Obstructive sleep apenia	OSA
Rule out	r/o
Anticoagulation	Antico-agx

List of medications commonly used

Brand	(Generic) Indication
Abilify	(Aripiprazole) Antipsychotic
Actonel	(Risedronate) Osteoporosis agent
Actos	(Pioglitazone) Antidiabetic
Advair	(Fluticasone + Salmeterol) Antiasthmatic
Aldactone	(Spirinolactone) <K+ sparing diuretic>
Allegra-D	(Fexofenadine + Pseudoephedrine) Antihistamine/ Decongestant
Ambien	(Zolpidem) Hypnotic sedative
Amoxil	(Amoxicillin) Penicillin Antibiotic
Flexeril	(Cyclobenzaprine) Muscle relaxant
Aleve	(Naproxen) NSAID
Antivert	(Meclizine) Anti-vertigo agent
Aricept	(Donepezil) Antipsychotic/ Agent for Alzheimer's Dementia
Atarax	(Hydroxyzine) Antianxiety/ Antipruritic
Ativan	(Lorazepam) Antianxiety
Augmentin	(Amoxicillin/ Clavulanate) Penicillin antibiotic w/ penicillinase inhibitor
Avandia	(Rosiglitazone) Antidiabetic
Avelox	(Moxifloxacin) Fluoroquinolone antibiotic
Avodart	(Dutasteride) Prostate anti-inflammatory
Bactrim, Septra	(Sulfamethoxazole/Trimethoprim) Sulfonamide antibiotic
Bactroban	(Mupirocin) Antibacterial <topical ointment>
Benadryl	(Diphenhydramine) Antihistamine
Benicar	(Olmesartan) Antihypertensive
Bentyl	(Dicyclomine) GI antispasmotic
Boniva	(Ibandronate) Osteoporosis agent

BuSpar	(Buspirone) Antianxiety agent
Capzasin-HP	(Capsaicin cream) Arthritis pain relief
Cardizem	(Diltiazem) Antihypertensive/anginal <non-DHP CCB>
Cardura	(Doxazosin) Antihypertensive/ BPH Agent <alpha-1 antagonist>
Catapres	(Clonidine) Antihypertensive <central α2-agonist>
Ceftin	(Cefuroxime) Cephalosporin Antibiotic 2nd G
Celebrex	(Celecoxib) NSAID, selective for COX2
Celexa	(Citalopram) Antidepressant SSRI
Chantix	(Varenicline) Smoking Cessation Aid
Cialis	(Tadalafil) Erectile dysftn
Cipro	(Ciprofloxacin) Fluoroquinolone antibiotic
Cleocin	(Clindamycin) Antibiotic
Cogentin	(Benztropine Mesylate) Anti-Parkinson
Colchicine	(generic only) anti-inflammotary for gout
Combivent	(Ipratropium + Albuterol MDI) Antiasthmatic
Cordarone	(Amiodarone) Antiarrhythmic <class III>
Coreg	(Carvedilol) Antihypertensive <nonselective beta-blocker with alpha-1 blocker)
Coumadin	(Warfarin) Anticoagulant
Cozaar	(Losartan) Antihypertensive
Crestor	(Rosuvastatin) Antihyperlipidemic, high potency <HMG-CoA reductase inhibitor>
Cymbalta	(Duloxetine) Antidepressant SNRI
Deltasone	(Prednisone) Anti-inflammatory
Depakote	(Divalproex) Antiepileptic/Antipsychotic

Desyrel	(Trazadone) Antidepressant
Detrol	(Tolterodine) Urinary bladder modifier
Diflucan	(Fluconazole) Antifungal
Dilantin Kapseals	(Phenytoin) Antiepileptic
Dilaudid	(Hydromorphone) Analgesic
Diovan	(Valsartan) Antihypertensive
Ditropan	(Oxybutynin) Urinary bladder modifier
Drisdol	(Vitamin D, Ergocalciferol) Vitamin
DuoNeb	(Ipratropium + Albuterol soln) Antiasthmatic
Duragesic	(Fentanyl) Opioid Analgesic
Dyazide, Maxzide	(Triamtrene/ HCTZ) Diuretic <K+ sparing + thiazide diuretic>
Ecotrin	(Aspirin, enteric-coated) Blood Modifier <platelet inhibitor>
Effexor	(Venlafaxine) Antidepressant SNRI
Effient	(Prasurgel) antiplatelets, used similar to plavix.
Elavil	(Amitriptyline) Antidepressant TCA
Eliquis	(ApiXaban) inhibit Factor X, novel oral anticoagx
Estrace	(Estradiol) Estrogen hormone, gel/tab/patch/vaginal/IM
Evista	(Raloxifene) Osteoporosis agent
Flagyl	(Metronidazole) Antibacterial/ Antiprotozoal
Flomax	(Tamsulosin) for BPH <alpha 1-a selective blocker>
Flonase	(Fluticasone) Antiallergy
Flovent	(Fluticasone MDI) Antiasthmatic
Fosamax	(Alendronate) Osteoporosis agent
Glucophage	(Metformin) Antidiabetic
Glucotrol	(Glipizide) Antidiabetic

Glucovance	(Glyburide/ Metformin) Antidiabetic
Haldol	(Haloperidol) Antipsychotic
Humalog	(Insulin Lispro, rDNA origin) Anti-diabetic
Humulin N, Humulin R	(Regular insulin NPH, Regular insulin) Anti-diabetic
HydroDiuril	(Hydrochlorothiazide) Thiazide Diuretic
Hytrin	(Terazosin) Antihypertensive/BPH <beta-1 antagonist>
Hyzaar	(Losartan + HCT) Antihypertensive
Imdur	(Isosorbide mononitrate) Antianginal
Integrilin	(Eptifibatide), anti-platelets, used mainly in PCI. Blocks binding of fibrinogen & von Willebrand factor to glycoprotein IIb/IIIa receptor on platelet surface
Isordil	(Isosorbide dinonitrate) Antianginal
Isoptin	(Verapimil) Antihypertensive/ Antianginal
Januvia	(Sitagliptin) Antidiabetic
Keflex	(Cephalexin) Cephalosporin antibiotic
Kenalog	(Tiramcinolone Acetonide) Topical Corticosteroid
Keppra	(Levetiracetam) Anti-convulsant
Klonopin	(Clonazepam) Antiepileptic
Lamicatal	(Lamotrigine) Antiepileptic
Lanoxin	(Digoxin) Inotropic agent
Lantus	(Insulin Glargine) Anti-diabetic
Lasix	(Furosemide) Loop Diuretic
Levaquin	(Levofloxacin) Fluoroquinolone antibiotic
Lexapro	(Escitalopram) Antidepressant SSRI
Lioresal	(Baclofen) Muscle relaxant
Lipitor	(Atorvastatin) Antihyperlipidemic, high potency <HMG-CoA reductase

inhibitor>

Lopid	(Gemfibrozil) Antihyperlipidemic <activate PPARa>
Lopressor	(Metoprolol Tartrate) Antihypertensive < B blocker>
Lortab, Vicodin	(Hydrocodone w/ tylenol) Opioid Analgesic
Lotensin	(Benazepril) Antihypertensive <ACE Inhibitor>
Lotrisone	(Clotrimazole w/ Betamethasone) Topical Antifungal
Lovaza	(Omega-3 FAs) Antihyperlipidemic
Lyrica	(Pregabalin) Anti-convulsant/Antineuralgic
Macrodantin, Macrobid	(Nitrofurantoin) Antibacterial
Medrol	(Methylpredisolone) Anti-inflammatory
Methadose, Dolophine	(Methadone) Opioid Analgesic
Micronase	(Glyburide) Antidiabetic
Miralax	(Polyethylene Glycol 2250) Laxative
Mobic	(Meloxicam) NSAID, non-selective COX inhipitor
Motrin	(Ibuprofen) NSAID
MS Contin	(Morphine Sulfate) Opioid Analgesic, long acting
Mytussin AC, Robutussin AC	(Codeine Phosphate w/ Guaifenesin) Antitussive/Expectorant
Namenda	(Memantine) Agent for Alzheimer's Dementia
Nasacort AQ	(Triamcinolone) Antiallergy
Nasonex	(Mometasone) Antiallergy
Neurontin	(Gabapentin) Antiepileptic, for neuropathy as well.
Nexium	(Esomeprazole) PPI

Niaspan	(Niacin) Antihyperlipidemic <increase lipoprotein lipase activity>
Nitrostat	(Nitroglycerin) Antianginal
Nizoral	(Ketoconazole) Antifungal
Norvasc	(Amlopidine) Antihypertensive <DHP CCB>
Novolog	(Insulin Aspart, rDNA origin) Anti-diabetic
NuvaRing	(Etonogestrel & Ethinyl estradiol) Contraceptive
Nystop	(Nystatin) Antifungal Antibiotic
Omnicef	(Cefdinir) Cephalosporin antibiotic, PO 3rd G
Oraped	(Prednisolone) Anti-inflammatory
Othro-Cyclen, Sprintec	(Norgestimate & Ethinyl estradiol) Oral contraceptive
Ovral, Lo/Ovral, Ogestrel,	(Noregestrel & Ethinyl estradiol) Oral contraceptive
Oxycontin	(Oxycodone CR) Opioid Analgesic
OxyIR, Roxicodone	(Oxycodone IR) Opioid Analgesic
Pamelor	(Nortriptyline) Antidepressant TCA
Paxil	(Paroxetine) Antidepressant SSRI
Pepcid	(Famotadine) Anti-ulcer agent
Percocet	(Oxycodone w/ tylenol) Opioid Analgesic
Phenergan	(Promethazine) Anti-emetic
Plaquenil	(Hydroxychloroquine) Antimalarial
Plavix	(Clopidogrel) Platelet Inhibitor
Pradaxa	(Dabigatran) inhibit thrombin, novel anticoagx
Pravachol	(Pravastatin) Antihyperlipidemic <HMG-CoA reductase inhibitor>
Premarin	(Conjugated estrogens) Estrogen

	Hormone
Prilosec	(Omeprazole) Anti-ulcer agent
Procardia, Nifedical, Adalet	(Nifedipine) Antihypertensive/ Antianginal <DHP CCB>
Proscar	(Finasteride) Prostate anti-inflammatory
Protonix	(Pantoprazole) Anti-ulcer agent
Proventil, Ventolin, Proair	(Albuterol) Anti-asthmatic
Prozac	(Fluoxetine) Antidepressant SSRI
Pyridium	(Phenazopyridine) Urinary tract analgesic
Ranexa	(Ranolazine) 2nd line anti-anginal, unknown mechanism.
Reglan	(Metoclopramide) Anti-emetic
Remeron	(Mirtazapine) Antidepressant
Requip	(Ropinirole) Anti-Parkinson, restless leg syndrome
Risperdal	(Risperidone) Antipsychotic
Robaxin	(Methocarbamol) Muscle relaxant
Seroquel	(Quetiapine) Antipsychotic
Singulair	(Montelukast) Antiasthmatic
Soma	(Carisoprodol) Muscle relaxant
Spiriva	(Tiotropium) Antiasthmatic
Suboxone	(Buprenorphine w/ Naloxone) Agent for Opioid Dependence
Synthroid, Levothyroid	(Levothyroxine) Thyroid hormone
Tamiflu	(Oseltamavir) Antiviral
Temovate	(Clobetasol Proprionate) Topical Anti-inflammatory
Tessalon	(Benzonatate) Antitussive
Topamax	(Topiramate) Antiepileptic

Toprol-XL	(Metoprolol Succinate) Antihypertensive <selective beta-1 blocker>
Tricor	(Fenofibrate) Antihyperlipidemic (mainly TG)
Tussionex	(Clorpheniramine w/ Hydrocodone) Antitussive
Ultram, Ryzolt	(Tramadol HCl) Analgesic
Valium	(Diazepam) Antianxiety
Valtrex	(Valacyclovir) Antiviral
Veramyst	(Fluticasone) Antiallergy
Viagra	(Sildenafil) Erectile dysftn
Victosa	(Liraglutide) SQ meds for DMII & obesity, increase insulin
Vibramycin	(Doxycycline) Tetracycline antibiotic
Avelox	(Moxifloxacin) Fluoroquinolone antibiotic
Vivelle-Dot	(Estradiol) Hormonal replacement <topical>
Voltaren	(Diclofenac) NSAID
Wellbutrin	(Bupropion) Antidepressant
Xanax	(Alprazolam) Antianxiety
Xarelto	(RivaroXaban) inhibit Factor X, novel oral anticoagx.
Xopenex	(Levalbuterol) Antiasthmatic
Yasmin, Ocella	(Drospirenone & Ethinyl estradiol) Oral contraceptive
Zanaflex	(Tizanidine) Muscle relaxant
Zantac	(Ranitidine) Anti-ulcer agent
Zebeta	(Bisoprolol) Antihypertensive
Zestril	(Lisinopril) Antihypertensive <ACE Inhibitor>
Zetia	(Ezetimibe) Antihyperlipidemic <inhibits intestinal absorption of cholesterol>

Zithromax, Z pack	(Azithromycin) Macrolide Antibiotic
Zocor	(Simvastatin) Antihyperlipidemic <HMG-CoA reductase inhibitor>
Zoloft	(Sertraline) Antidepressant SSRI
Zosyn	(Piperacillin/tazobactam) Antibiotic
Zovirax	(Acyclovir) Antiviral
Zyloprim	(Allopurinol) Agent for gout
Zyprexa	(Olanzapine) Atypical Antipsychotic

References

1. Harrison's Principles of Internal Medicine, 18th edition. Dan L. Longo, Editor, Anthony S. Fauci, Editor, Dennis L. Kasper, Editor, Stephen L. Hauser, Editor, J. Larry Jameson, Editor, Joseph Loscalzo, Editor
2. Foster C, Misry NF, Peddi PF, Sharma S. The Washington Manual of Medical Therapeutics. 33rd edition. Department of Medicine, Washington University School of Medicine. Wolters Kluwer/Lippincott Williams & Wilkins; 2010.
3. Sabatine MS. Pocket Medicine (The Massachusetts General Hospital Handbook of Internal Medicine). Fourth Edition. Wolters Kluwer/Lippincott Williams & Wilkins; 2010.
4. Rodvold KA, McConeghy KW et al. Methicillin-Resistant Staphylococcus aureus Therapy: Past, Present, and Future. CID;2014(1):S20-27.
5. Foster C, Misry NF, Peddi PF, Sharma S. The Washington Manual of Medical Therapeutics. 33rd edition. Department of Medicine, Washington University School of Medicine. Wolters Kluwer/Lippincott Williams & Wilkins; 2010.
6. Surawicz CM, Brandt LJ, Binion DG et al. Guidelines for Diagnosis, Treatment, and Prevention of Clostridium difficile infections. The American Journal of Gastroenterology. 2013;108(4):478-498.
7. Momeni M, Crucitti M, De Kock M. Patient-controlled analgesia in the management of postoperative pain. Drugs. 2006;66(18):2321-37.
8. Sabatine MS. Pocket Medicine (The Massachusetts General Hospital Handbook of Internal Medicine). Fourth Edition. Wolters Kluwer/Lippincott Williams & Wilkins; 2010.
9. Birdwell BG, Herbers JE, Kroenke K. Evaluating chest pain. The patient's presentation style alters the physician's diagnostic approach. Arch Intern Med 1993; 153:1991.
10. Pavlik VN, Hyman DJ, Wendt JA, Orengo C. Association of a culturally defined syndrome (nervios) with chest pain and DSM-IV affective disorders in Hispanic patients referred for cardiac stress testing. Ethn Dis 2004; 14:505.
11. Challenging existing paradigms in ischemic heart disease: the NHBLI-sponsored women's ischemia syndrome evaluation (WISE). J Am Coll Cardiol 2006; 47:1S.
12. D'Antono B, Dupuis G, Fortin C, et al. Angina symptoms in men and women with stable coronary artery disease and evidence of exercise-induced myocardial perfusion defects. Am Heart J 2006; 151:813.
13. von Kodolitsch Y, Schwartz AG, Nienaber CA. Clinical prediction of acute aortic dissection. Arch Intern Med 2000; 160:2977.
14. McGee, S. Pulmonary embolism. In: Evidence based physical diagnosis, 2, Saunders Elsevier, 2007. p.365.
15. Marcus GM, Cohen J, Varosy PD, et al. The utility of gestures in patients with chest discomfort. Am J Med 2007; 120:83.
16. Davies HA, Jones DB, Rhodes J, Newcombe RG. Angina-like esophageal pain: differentiation from cardiac pain by history. J Clin Gastroenterol 1985; 7:477. DWORKEN HJ, BIEL FJ, MACHELLA TE. Supradiaphragmatic reference of pain from the colon. Gastroenterology 1952; 22:222.
17. Ryle JA. Visceral pain and referred pain. Lancet 1926; 1:895.
18. Selzer M, Spencer WA. Convergence of visceral and cutaneous afferent pathways in the lumbar spinal cord. Brain Res 1969; 14:331.
19. Purcell TB. Nonsurgical and extraperitoneal causes of abdominal pain. Emerg Med Clin North Am 1989; 7:721.
20. Saik RP, Greenburg AG, Farris JM, Peskin GW. Spectrum of cholangitis. Am J Surg 1975; 130:143.
21. Go VL, Everhart JE. Pancreatitis. In: Digestive diseases in the United States: Epidemiology and impact, Everhart JE (Ed), National Institutes of Health, National Institute of Diabetes and Digestive and Kidney Diseases. US Government Printing Office, Washington, DC 1994. p.693.
22. Talley NJ, Colin-Jones D, Koch KL, et al. Functional dyspepsia: A classification with guidelines for diagnosis and management. Gastroenterol Int 1992; 4:145.
23. Flanagin BA, Mitchell MT, Thistlethwaite WA, Alverdy JC. Diagnosis and treatment of atypical presentations of hiatal hernia following bariatric surgery. Obes Surg 2010; 20:386.
24. Beeson MS. Splenic infarct presenting as acute abdominal pain in an older patient. J Emerg Med 1996; 14:319.
25. Nores M, Phillips EH, Morgenstern L, Hiatt JR. The clinical spectrum of splenic infarction. Am Surg 1998; 64:182.
26. Franklin QJ, Compeggie M. Splenic syndrome in sickle cell trait: four case presentations and a review of the literature. Mil Med 1999; 164:230.
27. Görg C, Seifart U, Görg K. Acute, complete splenic infarction in cancer patient is associated with a fatal outcome. Abdom Imaging 2004; 29:224. Hung JJ, Hsu HS, Huang CS, Yang KY. Tracheoesophageal fistula and tracheo-subclavian artery fistula after tracheostomy. Eur J Cardiothorac Surg 2007; 32:676.
28. Komatsu T, Sowa T, Fujinaga T, et al. Tracheo-innominate artery fistula: two case reports and a clinical review. Ann Thorac Cardiovasc Surg 2013; 19:60.
29. Choudhary C, Bandyopadhyay D, Salman R, et al. Broncho-vascular fistulas from self-expanding metallic stents: A retrospective case review. Ann Thorac Med 2013; 8:116.
30. Savale L, Parrot A, Khalil A, et al. Cryptogenic hemoptysis: from a benign to a life-threatening pathologic vascular condition. Am J Respir Crit Care Med 2007; 175:1181.
31. Kuzucu A, Gürses I, Soysal O, et al. Dieulafoy's disease: a cause of massive hemoptysis that is probably underdiagnosed. Ann Thorac Surg 2005; 80:1126.
32. Kolb T, Gilbert C, Fishman EK, et al. Dieulafoy's disease of the bronchus. Am J Respir Crit Care Med 2012; 186:1191.
33. Muniappan A, Tapias LF, Butala P, et al. Surgical therapy of pulmonary aspergillomas: a 30-year North American experience. Ann Thorac Surg 2014; 97:432.

34. Farid S, Mohamed S, Devbhandari M, et al. Results of surgery for chronic pulmonary Aspergillosis, optimal antifungal therapy and proposed high risk factors for recurrence--a National Centre's experience. J Cardiothorac Surg 2013; 8:180.

35. Ahmed S, Mohammad WW, Hamid F, et al. The 2011 dengue haemorrhagic fever outbreak in Lahore - an account of clinical parameters and pattern of haemorrhagic complications. J Coll Physicians Surg Pak 2013; 23:463.

36. Sareli AE, Janssen WJ, Sterman D, et al. Clinical problem-solving. What's the connection? - A 26-year-old white man presented to our referral hospital with a 1-month history of persistent cough productive of white sputum, which was occasionally tinged with blood. N Engl J Med 2008; 358:626.

37. Drent M, Wessels S, Jacobs JA, Thijssen H. Association of diffuse alveolar haemorrhage with acquired vitamin K deficiency. Respiration 2000; 67:697.

38. Ikeda M, Tanaka H, Sadamatsu K. Diffuse alveolar hemorrhage as a complication of dual antiplatelet therapy for acute coronary syndrome. Cardiovasc Revasc Med 2011; 12:407.

39. Chen BC, Sheth NR, Dadzie KA, et al. Hemodialysis for the treatment of pulmonary hemorrhage from dabigatran overdose. Am J Kidney Dis 2013; 62:591.

40. Heck SL, Blom P, Berstad A. Accuracy and complications in computed tomography fluoroscopy-guided needle biopsies of lung masses. Eur Radiol 2006; 16:1387.

41. Choi JW, Park CM, Goo JM, et al. C-arm cone-beam CT-guided percutaneous transthoracic needle biopsy of small (≤ 20 mm) lung nodules: diagnostic accuracy and complications in 161 patients. AJR Am J Roentgenol 2012; 199:W322.

42. Lee SM, Park CM, Lee KH, et al. C-arm cone-beam CT-guided percutaneous transthoracic needle biopsy of lung nodules: clinical experience in 1108 patients. Radiology 2014; 271:291.

43. Augoulea A, Lambrinoudaki I, Christodoulakos G. Thoracic endometriosis syndrome. Respiration 2008; 75:113.

44. Sandler A, Gray R, Perry MC, et al. Paclitaxel-carboplatin alone or with bevacizumab for non-small-cell lung cancer. N Engl J Med 2006; 355:2542.

45. Cho YJ, Murgu SD, Colt HG. Bronchoscopy for bevacizumab-related hemoptysis. Lung Cancer 2007; 56:465.

46. Karlson-Stiber C, Höjer J, Sjöholm A, et al. Nitrogen dioxide pneumonitis in ice hockey players. J Intern Med 1996; 239:451.

47. Centers for Disease Control and Prevention (CDC). Exposure to nitrogen dioxide in an indoor ice arena - New Hampshire, 2011. MMWR Morb Mortal Wkly Rep 2012; 61:139. American College of Cardiology Foundation, American Heart Association, European Society of Cardiology, et al. Management of patients with atrial fibrillation (compilation of 2006 ACCF/AHA/ESC and 2011 ACCF/AHA/HRS recommendations): a report of the American College of Cardiology/American Heart Association Task Force on practice guidelines. Circulation 2013; 127:1916.

48. January CT, Wann LS, Alpert JS, et al. 2014 AHA/ACC/HRS guideline for the management of patients with atrial fibrillation: a report of the American College of Cardiology/American Heart Association Task Force on practice guidelines and the Heart Rhythm Society. Circulation 2014; 130:e199.

49. January CT, Wann LS, Alpert JS, et al. 2014 AHA/ACC/HRS guideline for the management of patients with atrial fibrillation: executive summary: a report of the American College of Cardiology/American Heart Association Task Force on practice guidelines and the Heart Rhythm Society. Circulation 2014; 130:2071.

50. Wyse DG, Van Gelder IC, Ellinor PT, et al. Lone atrial fibrillation: does it exist? J Am Coll Cardiol 2014; 63:1715.

51. Kopecky SL, Gersh BJ, McGoon MD, et al. The natural history of lone atrial fibrillation. A population-based study over three decades. N Engl J Med 1987; 317:669.

52. Brand FN, Abbott RD, Kannel WB, Wolf PA. Characteristics and prognosis of lone atrial fibrillation. 30-year follow-up in the Framingham Study. JAMA 1985; 254:3449.

53. Kannel WB, Abbott RD, Savage DD, McNamara PM. Epidemiologic features of chronic atrial fibrillation: the Framingham study. N Engl J Med 1982; 306:1018.

54. Lévy S, Maarek M, Coumel P, et al. Characterization of different subsets of atrial fibrillation in general practice in France: the ALFA study. The College of French Cardiologists. Circulation 1999; 99:3028.

55. Takahashi N, Seki A, Imataka K, Fujii J. Clinical features of paroxysmal atrial fibrillation. An observation of 94 patients. Jpn Heart J 1981; 22:143.

56. Clementy J, Dulhoste MN, Laiter C, et al. Flecainide acetate in the prevention of paroxysmal atrial fibrillation: a nine-month follow-up of more than 500 patients. Am J Cardiol 1992; 70:44A.

57. EVANS W, SWANN P. Lone auricular fibrillation. Br Heart J 1954; 16:189.

58. LAMB LE, POLLARD LW. ATRIAL FIBRILLATION IN FLYING PERSONNEL. Circulation 1964; 29:694.

59. Peter RH, Gracey JG, Beach TB. A clinical profile of idiopathic atrial fibrillation. A functional disorder of atrial rhythm. Ann Intern Med 1968; 68:1288.

60. Rostagno C, Bacci F, Martelli M, et al. Clinical course of lone atrial fibrillation since first symptomatic arrhythmic episode. Am J Cardiol 1995; 76:837. Sterns RH, Silver SM. Salt and water: read the package insert. QJM 2003; 96:549.

61. Rose BD, Post TW. Clinical Physiology of Acid-Base and Electrolyte Disorders, 5th ed, McGraw-Hill, New York 2001. p.441.

62. Lu KC, Hsu YJ, Chiu JS, et al. Effects of potassium supplementation on the recovery of thyrotoxic periodic paralysis. Am J Emerg Med 2004; 22:544.

63. McCowen KC, Malhotra A, Bistrian BR. Stress-induced hyperglycemia. Crit Care Clin 2001; 17:107. tension. J Appl Physiol Respir Environ Exerc Physiol 1984; 57:686.

64. Taguchi O, Kikuchi Y, Hida W, et al. Effects of bronchoconstriction and external resistive loading on the sensation of dyspnea. J Appl Physiol (1985) 1991; 71:2183.

65. Moy ML, Woodrow Weiss J, Sparrow D, et al. Quality of dyspnea in bronchoconstriction differs from external resistive loads. Am J Respir Crit Care Med 2000; 162:451.

66. Clark AL, Piepoli M, Coats AJ. Skeletal muscle and the control of ventilation on exercise: evidence for metabolic receptors. Eur J Clin Invest 1995; 25:299.

67. Clark A, Volterrani M, Swan JW, et al. Leg blood flow, metabolism and exercise capacity in chronic stable heart failure. Int J Cardiol 1996; 55:127.
68. Killian KJ, Leblanc P, Martin DH, et al. Exercise capacity and ventilatory, circulatory, and symptom limitation in patients with chronic airflow limitation. Am Rev Respir Dis 1992; 146:935.
69. Melzack R, Torgerson WS. On the language of pain. Anesthesiology 1971; 34:50.
70. Melzack R. The McGill Pain Questionnaire: major properties and scoring methods. Pain 1975; 1:277.
71. Hunter M, Philips C. The experience of headache pain--an assessment of the qualities of tension headache pain. Pain 1981; 10:209. Netea MG, Kullberg BJ, Van der Meer JW. Circulating cytokines as mediators of fever. Clin Infect Dis 2000; 31 Suppl 5:S178.
72. Blatteis CM, Sehic E, Li S. Pyrogen sensing and signaling: old views and new concepts. Clin Infect Dis 2000; 31 Suppl 5:S168.
73. Saper CB, Breder CD. The neurologic basis of fever. N Engl J Med 1994; 330:1880.
74. Mitchell, JD, Grocott, HP, Phillips-Bute, B, et al. Cytokine secretion after cardiac surgery and its relationship to postoperative fever. Cytokine 2007; 39:37.
75. Dauleh MI, Rahman S, Townell NH. Open versus laparoscopic cholecystectomy: a comparison of postoperative temperature. J R Coll Surg Edinb 1995; 40:116.
76. Clark JA, Bar-Yosef S, Anderson A, et al. Postoperative hyperthermia following off-pump versus on-pump coronary artery bypass surgery. J Cardiothorac Vasc Anesth 2005; 19:426.
77. Ghert M, Allen B, Davids J, et al. Increased postoperative febrile response in children with osteogenesis imperfecta. J Pediatr Orthop 2003; 23:261. Rocha-Singh KJ, Eisenhauer AC, Textor SC, et al. Atherosclerotic Peripheral Vascular Disease Symposium II: intervention for renal artery disease. Circulation 2008; 118:2873.
78. Bortman G, Sellanes M, Odell DS, et al. Discrepancy between pre- and post-transplant diagnosis of end-stage dilated cardiomyopathy. Am J Cardiol 1994; 74:921.
79. Marwick TH. The viable myocardium: epidemiology, detection, and clinical implications. Lancet 1998; 351:815.
80. Allman KC, Shaw LJ, Hachamovitch R, Udelson JE. Myocardial viability testing and impact of revascularization on prognosis in patients with coronary artery disease and left ventricular dysfunction: a meta-analysis. J Am Coll Cardiol 2002; 39:1151.
81. Repetto A, Dal Bello B, Pasotti M, et al. Coronary atherosclerosis in end-stage idiopathic dilated cardiomyopathy: an innocent bystander? Eur Heart J 2005; 26:1519.
82. Jessup M, Brozena S. Heart failure. N Engl J Med 2003; 348:2007.
83. Koelling TM, Aaronson KD, Cody RJ, et al. Prognostic significance of mitral regurgitation and tricuspid regurgitation in patients with left ventricular systolic dysfunction. Am Heart J 2002; 144:524.
84. Fonarow GC, Yancy CW, Hernandez AF, et al. Potential impact of optimal implementation of evidence-based heart failure therapies on mortality. Am Heart J 2011; 161:1024.
85. Willenheimer R, van Veldhuisen DJ, Silke B, et al. Effect on survival and hospitalization of initiating treatment for chronic heart failure with bisoprolol followed by enalapril, as compared with the opposite sequence: results of the randomized Cardiac Insufficiency Bisoprolol Study (CIBIS) III. Circulation 2005; 112:2426.
86. Sliwa K, Norton GR, Kone N, et al. Impact of initiating carvedilol before angiotensin-converting enzyme inhibitor therapy on cardiac function in newly diagnosed heart failure. J Am Coll Cardiol 2004; 44:1825.
87. Fang JC. Angiotensin-converting enzyme inhibitors or beta-blockers in heart failure: does it matter who goes first? Circulation 2005; 112:2380.
88. Bristow MR, Gilbert EM, Abraham WT, et al. Carvedilol produces dose-related improvements in left ventricular function and survival in subjects with chronic heart failure. MOCHA Investigators. Circulation 1996; 94:2807.
89. Wikstrand J, Hjalmarson A, Waagstein F, et al. Dose of metoprolol CR/XL and clinical outcomes in patients with heart failure: analysis of the experience in metoprolol CR/XL randomized intervention trial in chronic heart failure (MERIT-HF). J Am Coll Cardiol 2002; 40:491.
90. Faris R, Flather MD, Purcell H, et al. Diuretics for heart failure. Cochrane Database Syst Rev 2006; :CD003838.
91. Effect of enalapril on mortality and the development of heart failure in asymptomatic patients with reduced left ventricular ejection fractions. The SOLVD Investigattors. N Engl J Med 1992; 327:685.
92. Cohn JN, Johnson G, Ziesche S, et al. A comparison of enalapril with hydralazine-isosorbide dinitrate in the treatment of chronic congestive heart failure. N Engl J Med 1991; 325:303.
93. Effects of enalapril on mortality in severe congestive heart failure. Results of the Cooperative North Scandinavian Enalapril Survival Study (CONSENSUS). The CONSENSUS Trial Study Group. N Engl J Med 1987; 316:1429.
94. Effect of enalapril on survival in patients with reduced left ventricular ejection fractions and congestive heart failure. The SOLVD Investigators. N Engl J Med 1991; 325:293.
95. Flather MD, Yusuf S, Køber L, et al. Long-term ACE-inhibitor therapy in patients with heart failure or left-ventricular dysfunction: a systematic overview of data from individual patients. ACE-Inhibitor Myocardial Infarction Collaborative Group. Lancet 2000; 355:1575.
96. Kostis JB, Shelton BJ, Yusuf S, et al. Tolerability of enalapril initiation by patients with left ventricular dysfunction: results of the medication challenge phase of the Studies of Left Ventricular Dysfunction. Am Heart J 1994; 128:358.
97. Packer M, Poole-Wilson PA, Armstrong PW, et al. Comparative effects of low and high doses of the angiotensin-converting enzyme inhibitor, lisinopril, on morbidity and mortality in chronic heart failure. ATLAS Study Group. Circulation 1999; 100:2312.
98. Delahaye F, de Gevigney G. Is the optimal dose of angiotensin-converting enzyme inhibitors in patients with congestive heart failure definitely established? J Am Coll Cardiol 2000; 36:2096.
99. Brophy JM, Joseph L, Rouleau JL. Beta-blockers in congestive heart failure. A Bayesian meta-analysis. Ann Intern Med 2001; 134:550.
100. Effect of metoprolol CR/XL in chronic heart failure: Metoprolol CR/XL Randomised Intervention Trial in Congestive Heart Failure (MERIT-HF). Lancet 1999; 353:2001. Ahmed A, Rich MW, Fleg

JL, et al. Effects of digoxin on morbidity and mortality in diastolic heart failure: the ancillary digitalis investigation group trial. Circulation 2006; 114:397.

101. Digitalis Investigation Group. The effect of digoxin on mortality and morbidity in patients with heart failure. N Engl J Med 1997; 336:525.

102. ALLHAT Officers and Coordinators for the ALLHAT Collaborative Research Group. The Antihypertensive and Lipid-Lowering Treatment to Prevent Heart Attack Trial. Major outcomes in high-risk hypertensive patients randomized to angiotensin-converting enzyme inhibitor or calcium channel blocker vs diuretic: The Antihypertensive and Lipid-Lowering Treatment to Prevent Heart Attack Trial (ALLHAT). JAMA 2002; 288:2981.

103. Beckett NS, Peters R, Fletcher AE, et al. Treatment of hypertension in patients 80 years of age or older. N Engl J Med 2008; 358:1887.

104. Wachtell K, Bella JN, Rokkedal J, et al. Change in diastolic left ventricular filling after one year of antihypertensive treatment: The Losartan Intervention For Endpoint Reduction in Hypertension (LIFE) Study. Circulation 2002; 105:1071.

105. Klingbeil AU, Schneider M, Martus P, et al. A meta-analysis of the effects of treatment on left ventricular mass in essential hypertension. Am J Med 2003; 115:41.

106. Bonow RO, Udelson JE. Left ventricular diastolic dysfunction as a cause of congestive heart failure. Mechanisms and management. Ann Intern Med 1992; 117:502.

107. Brutsaert DL, Sys SU, Gillebert TC. Diastolic failure: pathophysiology and therapeutic implications. J Am Coll Cardiol 1993; 22:318.

108. Bergström A, Andersson B, Edner M, et al. Effect of carvedilol on diastolic function in patients with diastolic heart failure and preserved systolic function. Results of the Swedish Doppler-echocardiographic study (SWEDIC). Eur J Heart Fail 2004; 6:453.

109. Andersson B, Caidahl K, di Lenarda A, et al. Changes in early and late diastolic filling patterns induced by long-term adrenergic beta-blockade in patients with idiopathic dilated cardiomyopathy. Circulation 1996; 94:673.

110. Poulsen SH, Jensen SE, Egstrup K. Effects of long-term adrenergic beta-blockade on left ventricular diastolic filling in patients with acute myocardial infarction. Am Heart J 1999; 138:710.

111. Flather MD, Shibata MC, Coats AJ, et al. Randomized trial to determine the effect of nebivolol on mortality and cardiovascular hospital admission in elderly patients with heart failure (SENIORS). Eur Heart J 2005; 26:215. Khalid S, Murdoch R, Newlands A, et al. Transient receptor potential vanilloid 1 (TRPV1) antagonism in patients with refractory chronic cough: a double-blind randomized controlled trial. J Allergy Clin Immunol 2014; 134:56.

112. Morice A, Kastelik JA, Thompson RH. Gender differences in airway behaviour. Thorax 2000; 55:629.

113. Kastelik JA, Thompson RH, Aziz I, et al. Sex-related differences in cough reflex sensitivity in patients with chronic cough. Am J Respir Crit Care Med 2002; 166:961.

114. Morice AH, Kastelik JA. Cough. 1: Chronic cough in adults. Thorax 2003; 58:901.

115. Kastelik JA, Aziz I, Ojoo JC, et al. Investigation and management of chronic cough using a probability-based algorithm. Eur Respir J 2005; 25:235.

116. Irwin RS, Madison JM. The diagnosis and treatment of cough. N Engl J Med 2000; 343:1715.

117. Pratter MR, Bartter T, Akers S, DuBois J. An algorithmic approach to chronic cough. Ann Intern Med 1993; 119:977.

118. Mello CJ, Irwin RS, Curley FJ. Predictive values of the character, timing, and complications of chronic cough in diagnosing its cause. Arch Intern Med 1996; 156:997.

119. McGarvey LP, Heaney LG, Lawson JT, et al. Evaluation and outcome of patients with chronic non-productive cough using a comprehensive diagnostic protocol. Thorax 1998; 53:738.

120. Iyer VN, Lim KG. Chronic cough: an update. Mayo Clin Proc 2013; 88:1115.

121. Kwon NH, Oh MJ, Min TH, et al. Causes and clinical features of subacute cough. Chest 2006; 129:1142.

122. Birring SS. Controversies in the evaluation and management of chronic cough. Am J Respir Crit Care Med 2011; 183:708.

123. Patrick H, Patrick F. Chronic cough. Med Clin North Am 1995; 79:361.

124. Pratter MR, Bartter T, Lotano R. The role of sinus imaging in the treatment of chronic cough in adults. Chest 1999; 116:1287.

125. Holinger LD, Sanders AD. Chronic cough in infants and children: an update. Laryngoscope 1991; 101:596.

126. Corrao WM, Braman SS, Irwin RS. Chronic cough as the sole presenting manifestation of bronchial asthma. N Engl J Med 1979; 300:633.

127. Johnson D, Osborn LM. Cough variant asthma: a review of the clinical literature. J Asthma 1991; 28:85.

128. O'Connell EJ, Rojas AR, Sachs MI. Cough-type asthma: a review. Ann Allergy 1991; 66:278.

129. Nakajima T, Nishimura Y, Nishiuma T, et al. Characteristics of patients with chronic cough who developed classic asthma during the course of cough variant asthma: a longitudinal study. Respiration 2005; 72:606.

130. McFadden ER Jr. Exertional dyspnea and cough as preludes to acute attacks of bronchial asthma. N Engl J Med 1975; 292:555.

131. Niimi A, Matsumoto H, Mishima M. Eosinophilic airway disorders associated with chronic cough. Pulm Pharmacol Ther 2009; 22:114.

132. Oh MJ, Lee JY, Lee BJ, Choi DC. Exhaled nitric oxide measurement is useful for the exclusion of nonasthmatic eosinophilic bronchitis in patients with chronic cough. Chest 2008; 134:990.

133. Hahn PY, Morgenthaler TY, Lim KG. Use of exhaled nitric oxide in predicting response to inhaled corticosteroids for chronic cough. Mayo Clin Proc 2007; 82:1350.

134. Prieto L, Ferrer A, Ponce S, et al. Exhaled nitric oxide measurement is NOT useful for predicting the response to inhaled corticosteroids in subjects with chronic cough. Chest 2009; 136:816.

135. Poe RH, Kallay MC. Chronic cough and gastroesophageal reflux disease: experience with specific therapy for diagnosis and treatment. Chest 2003; 123:679. White CW, Wright CB, Doty DB, et al. Does visual interpretation of the coronary arteriogram predict the physiologic importance of a coronary stenosis? N Engl J Med 1984; 310:819.

136. Ringqvist I, Fisher LD, Mock M, et al. Prognostic value of angiographic indices of coronary artery disease from the Coronary Artery Surgery Study (CASS). J Clin Invest 1983; 71:1854.

137. Emond M, Mock MB, Davis KB, et al. Long-term survival of medically treated patients in the Coronary Artery Surgery Study (CASS) Registry. Circulation 1994; 90:2645.
138. Gibbons RJ, Abrams J, Chatterjee K, et al. ACC/AHA 2002 guideline update for the management of patients with chronic stable angina www.acc.org/qualityandscience/clinical/statements.htm (Accessed on August 24, 2006).
139. Teo KK, Yusuf S, Furberg CD. Effects of prophylactic antiarrhythmic drug therapy in acute myocardial infarction. An overview of results from randomized controlled trials. JAMA 1993; 270:1589.
140. Braunwald E. Mechanism of action of calcium-channel-blocking agents. N Engl J Med 1982; 307:1618.
141. Heidenreich PA, McDonald KM, Hastie T, et al. Meta-analysis of trials comparing beta-blockers, calcium antagonists, and nitrates for stable angina. JAMA 1999; 281:1927.
142. Emanuelsson H, Egstrup K, Nikus K, et al. Antianginal efficacy of the combination of felodipine-metoprolol 10/100 mg compared with each drug alone in patients with stable effort-induced angina pectoris: a multicenter parallel group study. The TRAFFIC Study Group. Am Heart J 1999; 137:854.
143. Chaitman BR. Ranolazine for the treatment of chronic angina and potential use in other cardiovascular conditions. Circulation 2006; 113:2462.
144. Abrams J, Thadani U. Therapy of stable angina pectoris: the uncomplicated patient. Circulation 2005; 112:e255.
145. Winniford MD, Jansen DE, Reynolds GA, et al. Cigarette smoking-induced coronary vasoconstriction in atherosclerotic coronary artery disease and prevention by calcium antagonists and nitroglycerin. Am J Cardiol 1987; 59:203.
146. Winniford MD, Wheelan KR, Kremers MS, et al. Smoking-induced coronary vasoconstriction in patients with atherosclerotic coronary artery disease: evidence for adrenergically mediated alterations in coronary artery tone. Circulation 1986; 73:662.
147. van den Heuvel AF, Dunselman PH, Kingma T, et al. Reduction of exercise-induced myocardial ischemia during add-on treatment with the angiotensin-converting enzyme inhibitor enalapril in patients with normal left ventricular function and optimal beta blockade. J Am Coll Cardiol 2001; 37:470. Arnold AL, Milner KA, Vaccarino V. Sex and race differences in electrocardiogram use (the National Hospital Ambulatory Medical Care Survey). Am J Cardiol 2001; 88:1037.
148. Seils DM, Friedman JY, Schulman KA. Sex differences in the referral process for invasive cardiac procedures. J Am Med Womens Assoc 2001; 56:151.
149. Polk DM, Naqvi TZ. Cardiovascular disease in women: sex differences in presentation, risk factors, and evaluation. Curr Cardiol Rep 2005; 7:166.
150. Bairey Merz CN, Shaw LJ, Reis SE, et al. Insights from the NHLBI-Sponsored Women's Ischemia Syndrome Evaluation (WISE) Study: Part II: gender differences in presentation, diagnosis, and outcome with regard to gender-based pathophysiology of atherosclerosis and macrovascular and microvascular coronary disease. J Am Coll Cardiol 2006; 47:S21.
151. Mieres JH, Gulati M, Bairey Merz N, et al. Role of noninvasive testing in the clinical evaluation of women with suspected ischemic heart disease: a consensus statement from the American Heart Association. Circulation 2014; 130:350.
152. Orencia A, Bailey K, Yawn BP, Kottke TE. Effect of gender on long-term outcome of angina pectoris and myocardial infarction/sudden unexpected death. JAMA 1993; 269:2392.
153. Kannel WB, Vokonas PS. Demographics of the prevalence, incidence, and management of coronary heart disease in the elderly and in women. Ann Epidemiol 1992; 2:5.
154. Lerner DJ, Kannel WB. Patterns of coronary heart disease morbidity and mortality in the sexes: a 26-year follow-up of the Framingham population. Am Heart J 1986; 111:383.
155. Mosca L, Linfante AH, Benjamin EJ, et al. National study of physician awareness and adherence to cardiovascular disease prevention guidelines. Circulation 2005; 111:499.
156. Wenger NK. You've come a long way, baby: cardiovascular health and disease in women: problems and prospects. Circulation 2004; 109:558.
157. Alter DA, Naylor CD, Austin PC, Tu JV. Biology or bias: practice patterns and long-term outcomes for men and women with acute myocardial infarction. J Am Coll Cardiol 2002; 39:1909.
158. Michos ED, Vasamreddy CR, Becker DM, et al. Women with a low Framingham risk score and a family history of premature coronary heart disease have a high prevalence of subclinical coronary atherosclerosis. Am Heart J 2005; 150:1276. Taylor BC, Wilt TJ, Welch HG. Impact of diastolic and systolic blood pressure on mortality: implications for the definition of "normal". J Gen Intern Med 2011; 26:685.
159. Ahmed ME, Walker JM, Beevers DG, Beevers M. Lack of difference between malignant and accelerated hypertension. Br Med J (Clin Res Ed) 1986; 292:235.
160. Severe symptomless hypertension. Lancet 1989; 2:1369.
161. O'Mailia JJ, Sander GE, Giles TD. Nifedipine-associated myocardial ischemia or infarction in the treatment of hypertensive urgencies. Ann Intern Med 1987; 107:185.
162. Grossman E, Messerli FH, Grodzicki T, Kowey P. Should a moratorium be placed on sublingual nifedipine capsules given for hypertensive emergencies and pseudoemergencies? JAMA 1996; 276:1328.
163. Forman JP, Stampfer MJ, Curhan GC. Diet and lifestyle risk factors associated with incident hypertension in women. JAMA 2009; 302:401.
164. Sonne-Holm S, Sørensen TI, Jensen G, Schnohr P. Independent effects of weight change and attained body weight on prevalence of arterial hypertension in obese and non-obese men. BMJ 1989; 299:767.
165. Staessen JA, Wang J, Bianchi G, Birkenhäger WH. Essential hypertension. Lancet 2003; 361:1629.
166. Wang NY, Young JH, Meoni LA, et al. Blood pressure change and risk of hypertension associated with parental hypertension: the Johns Hopkins Precursors Study. Arch Intern Med 2008; 168:643.
167. Carnethon MR, Evans NS, Church TS, et al. Joint associations of physical activity and aerobic fitness on the development of incident hypertension: coronary artery risk development in young adults. Hypertension 2010; 56:49.

168.   de Simone G, Devereux RB, Chinali M, et al. Risk factors for arterial hypertension in adults with initial optimal blood pressure: the Strong Heart Study. Hypertension 2006; 47:162. Colberg SR, Sigal RJ, Fernhall B, et al. Exercise and type 2 diabetes: the American College of Sports Medicine and the American Diabetes Association: joint position statement. Diabetes Care 2010; 33:e147.
169.   American Diabetes Association. Standards of medical care in diabetes--2014. Diabetes Care 2014; 37 Suppl 1:S14.
170.   Centers for Disease Control and Prevention (CDC). Dental visits among dentate adults with diabetes--United States, 1999 and 2004. MMWR Morb Mortal Wkly Rep 2005; 54:1181.
171.   Inoue M, Iwasaki M, Otani T, et al. Diabetes mellitus and the risk of cancer: results from a large-scale population-based cohort study in Japan. Arch Intern Med 2006; 166:1871.
172.   Stattin P, Björ O, Ferrari P, et al. Prospective study of hyperglycemia and cancer risk. Diabetes Care 2007; 30:561.
173.   Hemminki K, Li X, Sundquist J, Sundquist K. Risk of cancer following hospitalization for type 2 diabetes. Oncologist 2010; 15:548.
174.   Giovannucci E, Harlan DM, Archer MC, et al. Diabetes and cancer: a consensus report. Diabetes Care 2010; 33:1674.
175.   Larsson SC, Mantzoros CS, Wolk A. Diabetes mellitus and risk of breast cancer: a meta-analysis. Int J Cancer 2007; 121:856.
176.   Tsilidis KK, Kasimis JC, Lopez DS, et al. Type 2 diabetes and cancer: umbrella review of meta-analyses of observational studies. BMJ 2015; 350:g7607. Booth GL, Kapral MK, Fung K, Tu JV. Recent trends in cardiovascular complications among men and women with and without diabetes. Diabetes Care 2006; 29:32.
177.   Vamos EP, Bottle A, Edmonds ME, et al. Changes in the incidence of lower extremity amputations in individuals with and without diabetes in England between 2004 and 2008. Diabetes Care 2010; 33:2592.
178.   Pasquale LR, Kang JH, Manson JE, et al. Prospective study of type 2 diabetes mellitus and risk of primary open-angle glaucoma in women. Ophthalmology 2006; 113:1081.
179.   Obrosova IG, Chung SS, Kador PF. Diabetic cataracts: mechanisms and management. Diabetes Metab Res Rev 2010; 26:172.
180.   Centers for Disease Control and Prevention (CDC). Correctable visual impairment among persons with diabetes--United States, 1999-2004. MMWR Morb Mortal Wkly Rep 2006; 55:1169. Global Strategy for Asthma Management and Prevention, Global Initiative for Asthma (GINA). www.ginasthma.org (Accessed on January 30, 2015).
181.   Standards for the diagnosis and care of patients with chronic obstructive pulmonary disease. American Thoracic Society. Am J Respir Crit Care Med 1995; 152:S77.
182.   Siafakas NM, Vermeire P, Pride NB, et al. Optimal assessment and management of chronic obstructive pulmonary disease (COPD). The European Respiratory Society Task Force. Eur Respir J 1995; 8:1398.
183.   BTS guidelines for the management of chronic obstructive pulmonary disease. The COPD Guidelines Group of the Standards of Care Committee of the BTS. Thorax 1997; 52 Suppl 5:S1.
184.   Obstructive lung disease. Med Clin North Am 1990; 74:547.
185.   Rosenbloom J, Campbell EJ, Mumford R, et al. Biochemical/immunologic markers of emphysema. Ann N Y Acad Sci 1991; 624 Suppl:7.
186.   Petty TL, Silvers GW, Stanford RE. Mild emphysema is associated with reduced elastic recoil and increased lung size but NOT with air-flow limitation. Am Rev Respir Dis 1987; 136:867.
187.   O'Brien C, Guest PJ, Hill SL, Stockley RA. Physiological and radiological characterisation of patients diagnosed with chronic obstructive pulmonary disease in primary care. Thorax 2000; 55:635.
188.   Jeffery PK. Comparison of the structural and inflammatory features of COPD and asthma. Giles F. Filley Lecture. Chest 2000; 117:251S.
189.   Castaldi PJ, San José Estépar R, Mendoza CS, et al. Distinct quantitative computed tomography emphysema patterns are associated with physiology and function in smokers. Am J Respir Crit Care Med 2013; 188:1083.
190.   Hersh CP, Washko GR, Estépar RS, et al. Paired inspiratory-expiratory chest CT scans to assess for small airways disease in COPD. Respir Res 2013; 14:42.
191.   Estépar RS, Kinney GL, Black-Shinn JL, et al. Computed tomographic measures of pulmonary vascular morphology in smokers and their clinical implications. Am J Respir Crit Care Med 2013; 188:231.
192.   Aoshiba K, Nagai A. Differences in airway remodeling between asthma and chronic obstructive pulmonary disease. Clin Rev Allergy Immunol 2004; 27:35.
193.   Baraldo S, Turato G, Badin C, et al. Neutrophilic infiltration within the airway smooth muscle in patients with COPD. Thorax 2004; 59:308.
194.   Sutherland ER, Martin RJ. Airway inflammation in chronic obstructive pulmonary disease: comparisons with asthma. J Allergy Clin Immunol 2003; 112:819.
195.   Turato G, Zuin R, Miniati M, et al. Airway inflammation in severe chronic obstructive pulmonary disease: relationship with lung function and radiologic emphysema. Am J Respir Crit Care Med 2002; 166:105.
196.   Cosio MG, Saetta M, Agusti A. Immunologic aspects of chronic obstructive pulmonary disease. N Engl J Med 2009; 360:2445.
197.   Hogg JC. Pathophysiology of airflow limitation in chronic obstructive pulmonary disease. Lancet 2004; 364:709.
198.   Hogg JC, Chu F, Utokaparch S, et al. The nature of small-airway obstruction in chronic obstructive pulmonary disease. N Engl J Med 2004; 350:2645. Jia CE, Zhang HP, Lv Y, et al. The Asthma Control Test and Asthma Control Questionnaire for assessing asthma control: Systematic review and meta-analysis. J Allergy Clin Immunol 2013; 131:695.
199.   Rank MA, Bertram S, Wollan P, et al. Comparing the Asthma APGAR system and the Asthma Control Test™ in a multicenter primary care sample. Mayo Clin Proc 2014; 89:917.
200.   Osborne ML, Pedula KL, O'Hollaren M, et al. Assessing future need for acute care in adult asthmatics: the Profile of Asthma Risk Study: a prospective health maintenance organization-based study. Chest 2007; 132:1151.

201. Enright PL, Lebowitz MD, Cockroft DW. Physiologic measures: pulmonary function tests. Asthma outcome. Am J Respir Crit Care Med 1994; 149:S9.
202. Crapo RO. Pulmonary-function testing. N Engl J Med 1994; 331:25.
203. Pennock BE, Cottrell JJ, Rogers RM. Pulmonary function testing. What is 'normal'? Arch Intern Med 1983; 143:2123.
204. Irvin, CG, Eidelman, D. Airways mechanics in asthma. In: Rhinitis and Asthma, Holgate, S, Busse, W (Eds), Blackwell Scientific Publications, Boston 1995. Wunderink RG, Waterer GW. Clinical practice. Community-acquired pneumonia. N Engl J Med 2014; 370:543.
205. Musher DM, Thorner AR. Community-acquired pneumonia. N Engl J Med 2014; 371:1619.
206. American Thoracic Society, Infectious Diseases Society of America. Guidelines for the management of adults with hospital-acquired, ventilator-associated, and healthcare-associated pneumonia. Am J Respir Crit Care Med 2005; 171:388.
207. Fine MJ, Auble TE, Yealy DM, et al. A prediction rule to identify low-risk patients with community-acquired pneumonia. N Engl J Med 1997; 336:243.
208. Metlay JP, Fine MJ. Testing strategies in the initial management of patients with community-acquired pneumonia. Ann Intern Med 2003; 138:109.
209. Lim WS, van der Eerden MM, Laing R, et al. Defining community acquired pneumonia severity on presentation to hospital: an international derivation and validation study. Thorax 2003; 58:377.
210. Bauer TT, Ewig S, Marre R, et al. CRB-65 predicts death from community-acquired pneumonia. J Intern Med 2006; 260:93.
211. Marrie TJ, Shariatzadeh MR. Community-acquired pneumonia requiring admission to an intensive care unit: a descriptive study. Medicine (Baltimore) 2007; 86:103. Nishimura RA, Otto CM, Bonow RO, et al. 2014 AHA/ACC guideline for the management of patients with valvular heart disease: a report of the American College of Cardiology/American Heart Association Task Force on Practice Guidelines. J Am Coll Cardiol 2014; 63:e57.
212. Shively BK, Gurule FT, Roldan CA, et al. Diagnostic value of transesophageal compared with transthoracic echocardiography in infective endocarditis. J Am Coll Cardiol 1991; 18:391.
213. Irani WN, Grayburn PA, Afridi I. A negative transthoracic echocardiogram obviates the need for transesophageal echocardiography in patients with suspected native valve active infective endocarditis. Am J Cardiol 1996; 78:101.
214. Gould FK, Denning DW, Elliott TS, et al. Guidelines for the diagnosis and antibiotic treatment of endocarditis in adults: a report of the Working Party of the British Society for Antimicrobial Chemotherapy. J Antimicrob Chemother 2012; 67:269.
215. Muñoz P, Bouza E, Marín M, et al. Heart valves should NOT be routinely cultured. J Clin Microbiol 2008; 46:2897.
216. Lepidi H, Casalta JP, Fournier PE, et al. Quantitative histological examination of mechanical heart valves. Clin Infect Dis 2005; 40:655. Marrie TJ. Community-acquired pneumonia. Clin Infect Dis 1994; 18:501.
217. Metlay JP, Kapoor WN, Fine MJ. Does this patient have community-acquired pneumonia? Diagnosing pneumonia by history and physical examination. JAMA 1997; 278:1440.
218. Jartti A, Rauvala E, Kauma H, et al. Chest imaging findings in hospitalized patients with H1N1 influenza. Acta Radiol 2011; 52:297.
219. Hopstaken RM, Witbraad T, van Engelshoven JM, Dinant GJ. Inter-observer variation in the interpretation of chest radiographs for pneumonia in community-acquired lower respiratory tract infections. Clin Radiol 2004; 59:743.
220. Albaum MN, Hill LC, Murphy M, et al. Interobserver reliability of the chest radiograph in community-acquired pneumonia. PORT Investigators. Chest 1996; 110:343. Büller HR, Bethune C, BhaNOT S, et al. Factor XI antisense oligonucleotide for prevention of venous thrombosis. N Engl J Med 2015; 372:232.
221. Travers RJ, Shenoi RA, Kalathottukaren MT, et al. Nontoxic polyphosphate inhibitors reduce thrombosis while sparing hemostasis. Blood 2014; 124:3183.
222. McMillan A, Bratton DJ, Faria R, et al. Continuous positive airway pressure in older people with obstructive sleep apnoea syndrome (PREDICT): a 12-month, multicentre, randomised trial. Lancet Respir Med 2014; 2:804.
223. http://www.accessdata.fda.gov/drugsatfda_docs/label/2015/206316lbl.pdf (Accessed on January 09, 2015).
224. Giugliano RP, Ruff CT, Braunwald E, et al. Edoxaban versus warfarin in patients with atrial fibrillation. N Engl J Med 2013; 369:2093.
225. Hokusai-VTE Investigators, Büller HR, Décousus H, et al. Edoxaban versus warfarin for the treatment of symptomatic venous thromboembolism. N Engl J Med 2013; 369:1406. Annane D, Bellissant E, Cavaillon JM. Septic shock. Lancet 2005; 365:63.
226. Vincent JL, Opal SM, Marshall JC, Tracey KJ. Sepsis definitions: time for change. Lancet 2013; 381:774.
227. Marshall JC, Cook DJ, Christou NV, et al. Multiple organ dysfunction score: a reliable descriptor of a complex clinical outcome. Crit Care Med 1995; 23:1638.
228. Vincent JL, Bihari DJ, Suter PM, et al. The prevalence of nosocomial infection in intensive care units in Europe. Results of the European Prevalence of Infection in Intensive Care (EPIC) Study. EPIC International Advisory Committee. JAMA 1995; 274:639.
229. Sands KE, Bates DW, Lanken PN, et al. Epidemiology of sepsis syndrome in 8 academic medical centers. JAMA 1997; 278:234.
230. Bone RC, Fisher CJ Jr, Clemmer TP, et al. A controlled clinical trial of high-dose methylprednisolone in the treatment of severe sepsis and septic shock. N Engl J Med 1987; 317:653.
231. Ziegler EJ, Fisher CJ Jr, Sprung CL, et al. Treatment of gram-negative bacteriemia and septic shock with HA-1A human monoclonal antibody against endotoxin. A randomized, double-blind, placebo-controlled trial. The HA-1A Sepsis Study Group. N Engl J Med 1991; 324:429.
232. Abraham E, Wunderink R, Silverman H, et al. Efficacy and safety of monoclonal antibody to human tumor necrosis factor alpha in patients with sepsis syndrome. A randomized, controlled, double-blind, multicenter clinical trial. TNF-alpha MAb Sepsis Study Group. JAMA 1995; 273:934.
233. Dhainaut JF, Vincent JL, Richard C, et al. CDP571, a humanized antibody to human tumor necrosis factor-alpha: safety, pharmacokinetics, immune response, and influence of the antibody

on cytokine concentrations in patients with septic shock. CPD571 Sepsis Study Group. Crit Care Med 1995; 23:1461.

234. Jones GR, Lowes JA. The systemic inflammatory response syndrome as a predictor of bacteraemia and outcome from sepsis. QJM 1996; 89:515.

235. Martin GS, Mannino DM, Moss M. The effect of age on the development and outcome of adult sepsis. Crit Care Med 2006; 34:15.

236. Dremsizov T, Clermont G, Kellum JA, et al. Severe sepsis in community-acquired pneumonia: when does it happen, and do systemic inflammatory response syndrome criteria help predict course? Chest 2006; 129:968.

237. Netea MG, van der Meer JW. Immunodeficiency and genetic defects of pattern-recognition receptors. N Engl J Med 2011; 364:60.

238. Martin GS, Mannino DM, Eaton S, Moss M. The epidemiology of sepsis in the United States from 1979 through 2000. N Engl J Med 2003; 348:1546.

239. Elixhauser A, Friedman B, Stranges E. Septicemia in U.S. Hospitals, 2009. Agency for Healthcare Research and Quality, Rockville, MD http://www.hcup-us.ahrq.gov/reports/statbriefs/sb122.pdf (Accessed on February 15, 2013).

240. Walkey AJ, Wiener RS, Lindenauer PK. Utilization patterns and outcomes associated with central venous catheter in septic shock: a population-based study. Crit Care Med 2013; 41:1450.

241. Kaukonen KM, Bailey M, Suzuki S, et al. Mortality related to severe sepsis and septic shock among critically ill patients in Australia and New Zealand, 2000-2012. JAMA 2014; 311:1308.

242. Esper AM, Martin GS. Extending international sepsis epidemiology: the impact of organ dysfunction. Crit Care 2009; 13:120.

243. Blanco J, Muriel-Bombín A, Sagredo V, et al. Incidence, organ dysfunction and mortality in severe sepsis: a Spanish multicentre study. Crit Care 2008; 12:R158. Díaz GG, Alcaraz AC, Talavera JC, et al. Noninvasive positive-pressure ventilation to treat hypercapnic coma secondary to respiratory failure. Chest 2005; 127:952.

244. Scala R, Naldi M, Archinucci I, et al. Noninvasive positive pressure ventilation in patients with acute exacerbations of COPD and varying levels of consciousness. Chest 2005; 128:1657.

245. Squadrone E, Frigerio P, Fogliati C, et al. Noninvasive vs invasive ventilation in COPD patients with severe acute respiratory failure deemed to require ventilatory assistance. Intensive Care Med 2004; 30:1303.

246. Paus-Jenssen ES, Reid JK, Cockcroft DW, et al. The use of noninvasive ventilation in acute respiratory failure at a tertiary care center. Chest 2004; 126:165.

247. Mal S, McLeod S, Iansavichene A, et al. Effect of out-of-hospital noninvasive positive-pressure support ventilation in adult patients with severe respiratory distress: a systematic review and meta-analysis. Ann Emerg Med 2014; 63:600.

248. Goodacre S, Stevens JW, Pandor A, et al. Prehospital noninvasive ventilation for acute respiratory failure: systematic review, network meta-analysis, and individual patient data meta-analysis. Acad Emerg Med 2014; 21:960.

249. Nava S, Navalesi P, Conti G. Time of non-invasive ventilation. Intensive Care Med 2006; 32:361.

250. Collaborative Research Group of Noninvasive Mechanical Ventilation for Chronic Obstructive Pulmonary Disease. Early use of non-invasive positive pressure ventilation for acute exacerbations of chronic obstructive pulmonary disease: a multicentre randomized controlled trial. Chin Med J (Engl) 2005; 118:2034.

251. Ozsancak Ugurlu A, Sidhom SS, Khodabandeh A, et al. Use and outcomes of noninvasive positive pressure ventilation in acute care hospitals in Massachusetts. Chest 2014; 145:964. Metz A, Hebbard G. Nausea and vomiting in adults--a diagnostic approach. Aust Fam Physician 2007; 36:688.

252. Scorza K, Williams A, Phillips JD, Shaw J. Evaluation of nausea and vomiting. Am Fam Physician 2007; 76:76.

253. Brzana RJ, Koch KL. Gastroesophageal reflux disease presenting with intractable nausea. Ann Intern Med 1997; 126:704.

254. Carney CP, Andersen AE. Eating disorders. Guide to medical evaluation and complications. Psychiatr Clin North Am 1996; 19:657.

255. Tack J, Talley NJ, Camilleri M, et al. Functional gastrointestinal disorders. In: Rome III, The Functional Gastrointestinal Disorders, 3rd ed, Drossman DA, et al (Eds), Degnon Associates, McLean, VA 2006.

256. Moffet HL. Common infections in ambulatory patients. Ann Intern Med 1978; 89:743.

257. Carmeli Y, Samore M, Shoshany O, et al. Utility of clinical symptoms versus laboratory tests for evaluation of acute gastroenteritis. Dig Dis Sci 1996; 41:1749.

258. Apfel CC, Korttila K, Abdalla M, et al. A factorial trial of six interventions for the prevention of postoperative nausea and vomiting. N Engl J Med 2004; 350:2441.

259. Sullivan S. Cannabinoid hyperemesis. Can J Gastroenterol 2010; 24:284.

260. Soriano-Co M, Batke M, Cappell MS. The cannabis hyperemesis syndrome characterized by persistent nausea and vomiting, abdominal pain, and compulsive bathing associated with chronic marijuana use: a report of eight cases in the United States. Dig Dis Sci 2010; 55:3113. Ros E, Zambon D. Postcholecystectomy symptoms. A prospective study of gall stone patients before and two years after surgery. Gut 1987; 28:1500.

261. Wilson RG, Macintyre IM. Symptomatic outcome after laparoscopic cholecystectomy. Br J Surg 1993; 80:439.

262. Arlow FL, Dekovich AA, Priest RJ, Beher WT. Bile acid-mediated postcholecystectomy diarrhea. Arch Intern Med 1987; 147:1327.

263. Breuer NF, Jaekel S, Dommes P, Goebell H. Fecal bile acid excretion pattern in cholecystectomized patients. Dig Dis Sci 1986; 31:953.

264. Schiller LR. Chronic Diarrhea. Curr Treat Options Gastroenterol 2005; 8:259.

265. Bryant DA, Mintz ED, Puhr ND, et al. Colonic epithelial lymphocytosis associated with an epidemic of chronic diarrhea. Am J Surg Pathol 1996; 20:1102.

266. Janda RC, Conklin JL, Mitros FA, Parsonnet J. Multifocal colitis associated with an epidemic of chronic diarrhea. Gastroenterology 1991; 100:458.

267. Mintz ED, Weber JT, Guris D, et al. An outbreak of Brainerd diarrhea among travelers to the Galapagos Islands. J Infect Dis 1998; 177:1041.

313

268.   Osterholm MT, MacDonald KL, White KE, et al. An outbreak of a newly recognized chronic diarrhea syndrome associated with raw milk consumption. JAMA 1986; 256:484.
269.   Vugia DJ, Abbott S, Mintz ED, et al. A restaurant-associated outbreak of Brainerd diarrhea in California. Clin Infect Dis 2006; 43:62. Voderholzer WA, Schatke W, Mühldorfer BE, et al. Clinical response to dietary fiber treatment of chronic constipation. Am J Gastroenterol 1997; 92:95.
270.   Anti M, Pignataro G, Armuzzi A, et al. Water supplementation enhances the effect of high-fiber diet on stool frequency and laxative consumption in adult patients with functional constipation. Hepatogastroenterology 1998; 45:727.
271.   Lembo A, Camilleri M. Chronic constipation. N Engl J Med 2003; 349:1360.
272.   Bharucha AE, Pemberton JH, Locke GR 3rd. American Gastroenterological Association technical review on constipation. Gastroenterology 2013; 144:218.
273.   Ramkumar D, Rao SS. Efficacy and safety of traditional medical therapies for chronic constipation: systematic review. Am J Gastroenterol 2005; 100:936.
274.   American College of Gastroenterology Chronic Constipation Task Force. An evidence-based approach to the management of chronic constipation in North America. Am J Gastroenterol 2005; 100 Suppl 1:S1.
275.   Corazziari E, Badiali D, Bazzocchi G, et al. Long term efficacy, safety, and tolerability of low daily doses of isosmotic polyethylene glycol electrolyte balanced solution (PMF-100) in the treatment of functional chronic constipation. Gut 2000; 46:522.
276.   Dipalma JA, Cleveland MV, McGowan J, Herrera JL. A randomized, multicenter, placebo-controlled trial of polyethylene glycol laxative for chronic treatment of chronic constipation. Am J Gastroenterol 2007; 102:1436.
277.   Lee-Robichaud H, Thomas K, Morgan J, Nelson RL. Lactulose versus Polyethylene Glycol for Chronic Constipation. Cochrane Database Syst Rev 2010; :CD007570. Villanueva C, Colomo A, Bosch A, et al. Transfusion strategies for acute upper gastrointestinal bleeding. N Engl J Med 2013; 368:11.
278.   Qaseem A, Humphrey LL, Fitterman N, et al. Treatment of anemia in patients with heart disease: a clinical practice guideline from the American College of Physicians. Ann Intern Med 2013; 159:770.
279.   Kravetz D, Bosch J, Arderiu M, et al. Hemodynamic effects of blood volume restitution following a hemorrhage in rats with portal hypertension due to cirrhosis of the liver: influence of the extent of portal-systemic shunting. Hepatology 1989; 9:808.
280.   Cerqueira RM, Andrade L, Correia MR, et al. Risk factors for in-hospital mortality in cirrhotic patients with oesophageal variceal bleeding. Eur J Gastroenterol Hepatol 2012; 24:551.
281.   Krige JE, Kotze UK, Distiller G, et al. Predictive factors for rebleeding and death in alcoholic cirrhotic patients with acute variceal bleeding: a multivariate analysis. World J Surg 2009; 33:2127.
282.   McCormick PA, Jenkins SA, McIntyre N, Burroughs AK. Why portal hypertensive varices bleed and bleed: a hypothesis. Gut 1995; 36:100.
283.   Restellini S, Kherad O, Jairath V, et al. Red blood cell transfusion is associated with increased rebleeding in patients with nonvariceal upper gastrointestinal bleeding. Aliment Pharmacol Ther 2013; 37:316.
284.   Wolf AT, Wasan SK, Saltzman JR. Impact of anticoagulation on rebleeding following endoscopic therapy for nonvariceal upper gastrointestinal hemorrhage. Am J Gastroenterol 2007; 102:290.
285.   Maltz GS, Siegel JE, Carson JL. Hematologic management of gastrointestinal bleeding. Gastroenterol Clin North Am 2000; 29:169.
286.   ASGE Standards of Practice Committee, Anderson MA, Ben-Menachem T, et al. Management of antithrombotic agents for endoscopic procedures. Gastrointest Endosc 2009; 70:1060. Palmer ED. The vigorous diagnostic approach to upper-gastrointestinal tract hemorrhage. A 23-year prospective study of 1,400 patients. JAMA 1969; 207:1477.
287.   Richards RJ, Donica MB, Grayer D. Can the blood urea nitrogen/creatinine ratio distinguish upper from lower gastrointestinal bleeding? J Clin Gastroenterol 1990; 12:500.
288.   Jensen DM, Machicado GA. Diagnosis and treatment of severe hematochezia. The role of urgent colonoscopy after purge. Gastroenterology 1988; 95:1569.
289.   Zuckerman GR, Trellis DR, Sherman TM, Clouse RE. An objective measure of stool color for differentiating upper from lower gastrointestinal bleeding. Dig Dis Sci 1995; 40:1614.
290.   Wilcox CM, Alexander LN, Cotsonis G. A prospective characterization of upper gastrointestinal hemorrhage presenting with hematochezia. Am J Gastroenterol 1997; 92:231.
291.   Laine L, Shah A. Randomized trial of urgent vs. elective colonoscopy in patients hospitalized with lower GI bleeding. Am J Gastroenterol 2010; 105:2636.
292.   Srygley FD, Gerardo CJ, Tran T, Fisher DA. Does this patient have a severe upper gastrointestinal bleed? JAMA 2012; 307:1072.
293.   Jensen DM, Machicado GA, Jutabha R, Kovacs TO. Urgent colonoscopy for the diagnosis and treatment of severe diverticular hemorrhage. N Engl J Med 2000; 342:78.
294.   Davila RE, Rajan E, Adler DG, et al. ASGE Guideline: the role of endoscopy in the patient with lower-GI bleeding. Gastrointest Endosc 2005; 62:656.
295.   Lewis JD, Brown A, Localio AR, Schwartz JS. Initial evaluation of rectal bleeding in young persons: a cost-effectiveness analysis. Ann Intern Med 2002; 136:99.
296.   Kollef MH, O'Brien JD, Zuckerman GR, Shannon W. BLEED: a classification tool to predict outcomes in patients with acute upper and lower gastrointestinal hemorrhage. Crit Care Med 1997; 25:1125.
297.   Velayos FS, Williamson A, Sousa KH, et al. Early predictors of severe lower gastrointestinal bleeding and adverse outcomes: a prospective study. Clin Gastroenterol Hepatol 2004; 2:485.
298.   Strate LL, Orav EJ, Syngal S. Early predictors of severity in acute lower intestinal tract bleeding. Arch Intern Med 2003; 163:838.
299.   Das A, Ben-Menachem T, Cooper GS, et al. Prediction of outcome in acute lower-gastrointestinal haemorrhage based on an artificial neural network: internal and external validation of a predictive model. Lancet 2003; 362:1261.
300.   Baradarian R, Ramdhaney S, Chapalamadugu R, et al. Early intensive resuscitation of patients with upper gastrointestinal bleeding decreases mortality. Am J Gastroenterol 2004; 99:619.

314

301. Villanueva C, Colomo A, Bosch A, et al. Transfusion strategies for acute upper gastrointestinal bleeding. N Engl J Med 2013; 368:11. Mandell LA, Wunderink RG, Anzueto A, et al. Infectious Diseases Society of America/American Thoracic Society consensus guidelines on the management of community-acquired pneumonia in adults. Clin Infect Dis 2007; 44 Suppl 2:S27.
302. Marrie TJ, Poulin-Costello M, Beecroft MD, Herman-Gnjidic Z. Etiology of community-acquired pneumonia treated in an ambulatory setting. Respir Med 2005; 99:60. Drlica K, Zhao X. DNA gyrase, topoisomerase IV, and the 4-quinolones. Microbiol Mol Biol Rev 1997; 61:377.
303. Hooper DC. Mechanisms of fluoroquinolone resistance. Drug Resist Updat 1999; 2:38.
304. Neugut AI, Ghatak AT, Miller RL. Anaphylaxis in the United States: an investigation into its epidemiology. Arch Intern Med. 2001;161:15-21.
305. Colgan R, Powers JH. Appropriate antimicrobial prescribing: approaches that limit antibiotic resistance. Am Fam Physician. 2001;64:999-1004.
306. Gonzalez LS 3rd. Aminoglycosides: a practical review. Am Fam Physician. 1998;58:1811-1820.
307. File TM. Community-acquired pneumonia. Lancet. 2003;362:1991-2001.
308. Siempos II, Dimopolous G, Falagas, ME. Meta-analyses on the prevention and treatment of respiratory tract infections. Infect Dis Clin North Am. 2009;23:331-353.
309. Farrell DJ, Jenkins SG. Distribution across the USA of macrolide resistance and macrolide resistance mechanisms among Streptococus pneumoniae isolates collected from patients with respiratory tract infections: PROTEKT US 2001-2002. J Antimicrob Chemother. 2004;54(Suppl 1):i17-22.
310. Brown SD, Farrell DJ. Antibacterial susceptibility among Streptococcus pneumoniae isolated from paediatric and adult patients as part of the PROTEKT US study in 2001-2002. J Antimicrob Chemother. 2004;54(Suppl S1):i23-9. Chartier C, Grosshans E. Erysipelas: an update. Int J Dermatol 1996; 35:779.
311. Barzilai A, Choen HA. Isolation of group A streptococci from children with perianal cellulitis and from their siblings. Pediatr Infect Dis J 1998; 17:358.
312. Thorsteinsdottir B, Tleyjeh IM, Baddour LM. Abdominal wall cellulitis in the morbidly obese. Scand J Infect Dis 2005; 37:605.
313. Dupuy A, Benchikhi H, Roujeau JC, et al. Risk factors for erysipelas of the leg (cellulitis): case-control study. BMJ 1999; 318:1591.
314. McNamara DR, Tleyjeh IM, Berbari EF, et al. A predictive model of recurrent lower extremity cellulitis in a population-based cohort. Arch Intern Med 2007; 167:709. Digby JM, Kersley JB. Pyogenic non-tuberculous spinal infection: an analysis of thirty cases. J Bone Joint Surg Br. Feb 1979;61(1):47-55. [Medline].
315. Böhm E, Josten C. What's new in exogenous osteomyelitis?. Pathol Res Pract. Feb 1992;188(1-2):254-8.[Medline].
316. Laughlin RT, Reeve F, Wright DG, Mader JT, Calhoun JH. Calcaneal osteomyelitis caused by nail puncture wounds. Foot Ankle Int. Sep 1997;18(9):575-7. [Medline].
317. Mader JT, Cripps MW, Calhoun JH. Adult posttraumatic osteomyelitis of the tibia. Clin Orthop Relat Res. Mar 1999;(360):14-21. [Medline].
318. Roesgen M, Hierholzer G, Hax PM. Post-traumatic osteomyelitis. Pathophysiology and management. Arch Orthop Trauma Surg. 1989;108(1):1-9. [Medline].
319. Weber EJ. Plantar puncture wounds: a survey to determine the incidence of infection. J Accid Emerg Med. Jul 1996;13(4):274-7. [Medline]. Jackson SL, Boyko EJ, Scholes D, et al. Predictors of urinary tract infection after menopause: a prospective study. Am J Med 2004; 117:903.
320. Czaja CA, Scholes D, Hooton TM, Stamm WE. Population-based epidemiologic analysis of acute pyelonephritis. Clin Infect Dis 2007; 45:273.
321. Echols RM, Tosiello RL, Haverstock DC, Tice AD. Demographic, clinical, and treatment parameters influencing the outcome of acute cystitis. Clin Infect Dis 1999; 29:113.
322. Hooton TM. Clinical practice. Uncomplicated urinary tract infection. N Engl J Med 2012; 366:1028.
323. Gupta K, Trautner B. In the clinic. Urinary tract infection. Ann Intern Med 2012; 156:ITC3.
324. Hooton TM, Roberts PL, Cox ME, Stapleton AE. Voided midstream urine culture and acute cystitis in premenopausal women. N Engl J Med 2013; 369:1883.
325. Kahlmeter G. Prevalence and antimicrobial susceptibility of pathogens in uncomplicated cystitis in Europe. The ECO.SENS study. Int J Antimicrob Agents 2003; 22 Suppl 2:49.
326. Kahlmeter G, ECO.SENS. An international survey of the antimicrobial susceptibility of pathogens from uncomplicated urinary tract infections: the ECO.SENS Project. J Antimicrob Chemother 2003; 51:69.
327. Naber KG, Schito G, Botto H, et al. Surveillance study in Europe and Brazil on clinical aspects and Antimicrobial Resistance Epidemiology in Females with Cystitis (ARESC): implications for empiric therapy. Eur Urol 2008; 54:1164. Payen D, de Pont AC, Sakr Y, et al. A positive fluid balance is associated with a worse outcome in patients with acute renal failure. Crit Care 2008; 12:R74.
328. Bouchard J, Soroko SB, Chertow GM, et al. Fluid accumulation, survival and recovery of kidney function in critically ill patients with acute kidney injury. Kidney Int 2009; 76:422.
329. Kraut JA, Kurtz I. Use of base in the treatment of severe acidemic states. Am J Kidney Dis 2001; 38:703.
330. Marsh JD, Margolis TI, Kim D. Mechanism of diminished contractile response to catecholamines during acidosis. Am J Physiol 1988; 254:H20.
331. Mitchell JH, Wildenthal K, Johnson RL Jr. The effects of acid-base disturbances on cardiovascular and pulmonary function. Kidney Int 1972; 1:375.
332. Teplinsky K, O'Toole M, Olman M, et al. Effect of lactic acidosis on canine hemodynamics and left ventricular function. Am J Physiol 1990; 258:H1193.
333. Orchard CH, Kentish JC. Effects of changes of pH on the contractile function of cardiac muscle. Am J Physiol 1990; 258:C967.
334. Mathieu D, Neviere R, Billard V, et al. Effects of bicarbonate therapy on hemodynamics and tissue oxygenation in patients with lactic acidosis: a prospective, controlled clinical study. Crit Care Med 1991; 19:1352.
335. Orchard CH, Cingolani HE. Acidosis and arrhythmias in cardiac muscle. Cardiovasc Res 1994; 28:1312.